Knowing and Understanding ADHD in the Light of New Scientific Evidence and Research Suggestion

Edited by Marco Carotenuto and Giuditta Bargiacchi

Published in London, United Kingdom

Knowing and Understanding ADHD in the Light of New Scientific Evidence and Research Suggestion
http://dx.doi.org/10.5772/intechopen.1008078
Edited by Marco Carotenuto and Giuditta Bargiacchi

Contributors
Alessandra Carta, Fatimah Saeed Alahmari, Giuditta Bargiacchi, Giulia Santangelo, Jamuna Das, Jitendriya Biswal, Khoulod Mohamed, Madeeha Kamal, Marco Carotenuto, Martina Gnazzo, Selman Yildirim, Stefano Sotgiu, Valentina Baldini, Vanna Cavassa

First published in London, United Kingdom, 2025 by IntechOpen
IntechOpen is the global imprint of INTECHOPEN LIMITED, registered in England and Wales, registration number: 11086078, 167-169 Great Portland Street, London, W1W 5PF, United Kingdom

For EU product safety concerns: IN TECH d.o.o., Prolaz Marije Krucifikse Kozulić 3, 51000 Rijeka, Croatia, info@intechopen.com or visit our website at intechopen.com.

British Library Cataloguing-in-Publication Data
A catalogue record for this book is available from the British Library

Knowing and Understanding ADHD in the Light of New Scientific Evidence and Research Suggestion
Edited by Marco Carotenuto and Giuditta Bargiacchi
p. cm.

This title is part of the Nervous System and Mental Health Book Series, Volume 2
Series Editor: Toshikazu Shinba

Print ISBN 978-1-83634-221-2
Online ISBN 978-1-83634-220-5
eBook (PDF) ISBN 978-1-83634-222-9
ISSN 3050-2985

If disposing of this product, please recycle the paper responsibly.

IntechOpen Book Series

Nervous System and Mental Health

Volume 2

Aims and Scope of the Series

Mental health is frequently linked to the nervous system. Conversely, disturbances in the nervous system often lead to mental health problems. However, this linkage is not as clear as it is commonly accepted. Mental health is usually described using subjective terms, which are based on psychological and psychiatric symptomatology. Diagnosis of a mental illness is made through the presence of the subjective symptoms characterizing the illness.

On the other hand, the nervous system has been deeply investigated using objective measures, including molecular, genetic, imaging, pharmacological and physiological ones. It is essential to combine objective views of the nervous system with subjective perspectives on mental health to develop an integrative approach to understanding human cognitive functions and achieving overall well-being. In this book series, experts in various fields of the nervous system and mental health will present their views on these challenging topics.

Meet the Series Editor

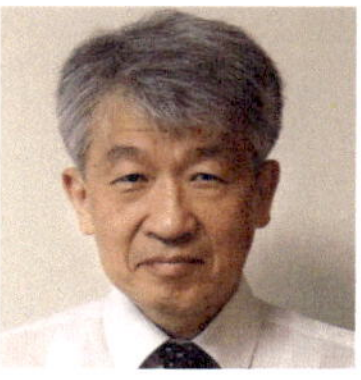

Dr. Toshikazu Shinba is a psychiatrist and neuroscientist who has been working in both clinical and basic research fields. He has been affiliated with the Tokyo Institute of Psychiatry, Department of Neurophysiology and Stress Disorders Project, and now works as a psychiatrist at Shizuoka Saiseikai General Hospital, Department of Psychiatry. The primary focus of his research is the electrophysiological analysis of attention and arousal in both humans and rodents. In clinical research, EEG, heart rate variability and skin conductance have been measured in mental disorders and arousal/consciousness disturbances. In basic research, single neuronal firing and EEG recordings have been assessed in rats. His research interests cover physiological rhythms related to attention, arousal, and consciousness in both the central and peripheral nervous systems, with a focus on understanding mental states.

Meet the Volume Editor

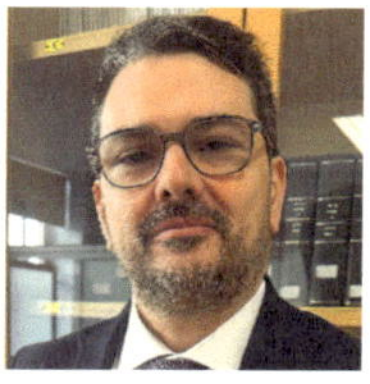

Marco Carotenuto, M. D., Ph.D., M. S., is a Full Professor of Child Neuropsychiatry at the University of Campania "Luigi Vanvitelli" in Italy, where he also directs the Child Neuropsychiatry Unit. He earned his medical degree there in 2000, specialized in Child Neuropsychiatry in 2005 after completing clinical training in the UK, and obtained a Ph.D. in Behavioral Sciences and Learning Disorders in 2008. Appointed Full Professor in 2018, he leads in both academia and clinical practice. Since 2022, he has served as President of the National Commission for Neurotherapy and Psychomotor Therapy in Developmental Age (TNPEE) and directs the School of Specialization in Child Neuropsychiatry. Author of over 300 publications, his work focuses on autism, sleep disturbances, headaches, epilepsy, and neurocognitive rehabilitation in children.

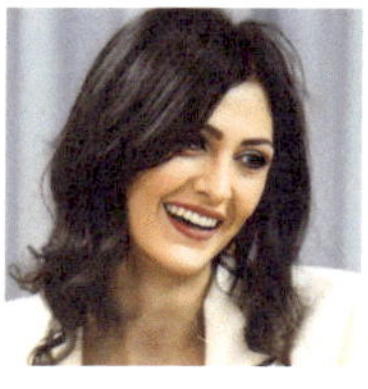

Dr. Giuditta Bargiacchi graduated in Medicine from the University of Campania "Luigi Vanvitelli" in Italy and is a final-year registrar in Child and Adolescent Neuropsychiatry. During her training, she has gained extensive hospital-based clinical experience, with a strong focus on neurodevelopmental disorders. Her main scientific interests center on the genetic and neurobiological bases of rare variants associated with neuropsychomotor impairment, as well as the clinical management of epilepsy in childhood and adolescence. She is the author of several peer-reviewed publications and has presented her research at national and international conferences, contributing to the understanding of complex neurodevelopmental conditions. Alongside her clinical and research commitments, Dr. Bargiacchi is actively involved in medical education and participates in important awareness and information campaigns across the Campania region. Dr. Bargiacchi is actively involved in medical education and is currently pursuing a Master's degree in Experimental and Clinical Neuropsychoneuroimmunology at the University of Rome "Tor Vergata," with a focus on the pharmacological modulation of neuroinflammation as a promising therapeutic approach for autism spectrum disorders.

Contents

Preface **XIII**

Section 1
Reconceptualising ADHD: Complexity, Comorbidities and Foundational Insights **1**

Chapter 1 **3**
Introductory Chapter: Rethinking ADHD in the Age of Multidimensional Science
by Marco Carotenuto

Chapter 2 **7**
ADHD in School Age Children: Overview
by Fatimah Saeed Alahmari

Chapter 3 **31**
Perspective Chapter: The Impact of Circadian Rhythm Dysregulation in the Treatment Resistance and Medication Efficacy of ADHD across the Lifespan
by Alessandra Carta, Vanna Cavassa and Stefano Sotgiu

Chapter 4 **51**
Sleep and ADHD
by Martina Gnazzo, Valentina Baldini, Giulia Santangelo, Giuditta Bargiacchi and Marco Carotenuto

Section 2
Innovation and Translational Pathways in ADHD Diagnosis and Care **61**

Chapter 5 **63**
ADHD Co-Occurring Conditions: A Multidisciplinary Approach
by Jamuna Das and Jitendriya Biswal

Chapter 6 **87**
Updates on ADHD in Children and Adolescents: Approach to Diagnosis and Management
by Madeeha Kamal and Khoulod Mohamed

Chapter 7 **103**
The Role of Artificial Intelligence in ADHD Diagnosis and Treatment: A New Frontier in Neurotechnology
by Selman Yildirim

Preface

Attention-Deficit/Hyperactivity Disorder (ADHD) is a condition that has been the subject of ongoing debate and discovery, particularly with the growing recognition of adult cases and the emergence of previously overlooked signs and symptoms in women. This diversity and complexity make ADHD a significant health problem, regardless of age and gender. While numerous books and articles have attempted to explain its symptoms, causes, and treatments, "Knowing and Understanding ADHD in the Light of New Scientific Evidence and Research Suggestions" offers a unique perspective on this multifaceted condition. This volume was conceived with the idea that ADHD cannot be fully understood through a single lens. Instead, it should be approached as a multifaceted condition, shaped not only by neurobiology but also by behaviour, environment, learning contexts, and even cultural shifts. Many of the chapters included here revisit topics already well-known in the clinical field, but they do so from fresh perspectives, highlighting new correlations and challenging established assumptions. Others introduce innovative areas of research, such as the role of sleep regulation, the contribution of neuroinflammatory processes, or the impact of technology and digital environments on attention and executive functions. In particular, the neurobiological view is privileged as a summa omnia of current knowledge, while also offering a highly dynamic perspective. This volume aims to offer diverse reflections on seemingly familiar topics, enriching, rather than weakening, existing knowledge. Academic conceptualisations or rigid diagnostic criteria may not always accurately reflect the patient's reality, especially during the developmental years. The relevance of this book lies in its emphasis on translating evidence into personalised approaches. It recognises that ADHD is not a universal condition and that therapeutic strategies should reflect this diversity. The academic description of this disorder is general, but only the clinician can understand the specifics of each patient. Individualised interventions, based on the recognition of individual differences, offer the most promising path. Combining the latest scientific discoveries with forward-looking research insights, this book provides readers with practical insights and conceptual tools to rethink clinical practice and educational strategies, instilling hope and reassurance. The goal of this book is not only to summarise knowledge, but also to stimulate dialogue and promote innovation. Our goal is to inspire clinicians, teachers, researchers, and families to adopt a broader and more nuanced view of ADHD, embracing its complexity while always keeping the individual at the center of care and support. By doing so, we can always emerge victorious from the disorder, and we hope that this work will motivate and engage our readers in this important mission.

Marco Carotenuto and Giuditta Bargiacchi
Child Neuropsychiatry,
Department of Mental and Physical Health and Preventive Medicine,
University of Campania "Luigi Vanvitelli",
Caserta, Italy

Section 1

Reconceptualising ADHD: Complexity, Comorbidities and Foundational Insights

Chapter 1

Introductory Chapter: Rethinking ADHD in the Age of Multidimensional Science

Marco Carotenuto

1. Introduction

Attention-Deficit/Hyperactivity Disorder (ADHD) is a widespread and complex neurodevelopmental condition characterised by persistent patterns of inattention, hyperactivity, and impulsivity that significantly impair functioning in multiple significant areas of the patient's life, regardless of age and gender [1]. Symptoms typically begin during childhood, but symptoms often persist into adolescence and adulthood, affecting approximately 5–7% of children and approximately 2.5–3% of adults globally [2]. And late or very late diagnoses should not be overlooked, even in individuals who appear to be well-integrated into a seemingly regular life, although ADHD is frequently associated with other physical and psychiatric disorders, such as neurodevelopmental, conduct, anxiety, and mood disorders [3].

2. Aetiology and pathophysiology

Now that the sterile debate over the non-existence of the disorder, stigmatised by the medicalisation of normal developmental behaviours, has been abandoned, intensive research conducted in recent decades has revealed that ADHD is rooted in neurobiological abnormalities, particularly in the brain circuits involved in executive functions, self-regulation, and reward and motivation processing. These include reduced structural and functional connectivity in the prefrontal cortex, basal ganglia, and anterior cingulate cortex, along with imbalances in the dopamine and norepinephrine signalling pathways [4, 5]. Specifically, ADHD should be characterised as a sort of hyperdopaminergic syndrome. Additionally, disturbances in circadian rhythms contribute to sleep dysregulation and metabolic dysfunction, further exacerbating symptom severity [4, 6].

ADHD was once considered a disorder whose aetiology was more influenced by epigenetic factors than genetic ones.

Genetic factors, however, account for approximately 70–80% of the variance in ADHD risk, while non-shared environmental influences, such as prenatal exposures or brain injuries, account for the remainder [7] .

Emerging neuroimaging techniques have significantly improved our understanding. For example, dynamic functional connectivity analyses suggest increased temporal instability within large-scale networks in individuals with ADHD, offering a plausible link to behavioural variability and attention deficits.

3. Heterogeneity across development

ADHD is not a single, monolithic disorder but encompasses multiple presentations, including predominantly inattentive, hyperactive-impulsive, and combined types. These diverse trajectories suggest that it is a neurobiological syndrome, still observed only in its most obvious clinical manifestations. While many children experience remission or attenuation of symptoms over time, a significant percentage continue to meet full diagnostic criteria into adulthood. Symptoms often present differently based on age and gender: for example, girls and women may be underdiagnosed in childhood due to more subtle internalising symptoms compared to the more obvious hyperactivity observed in boys. Above all, motor hyperactivity tends to subside in most individuals from adolescence onward, while strategies are developed to be or appear adequately attentive. Only the impulsive component never abandons the patient, as it is a true cognitive style intrinsically constitutive of the individual who develops ADHD symptoms [8].

4. Clinical and societal impact

ADHD poses significant challenges—not only for the affected individuals but also for families, educational systems, and healthcare infrastructure. Patients with ADHD are at increased risk for co-occurring mental health conditions (e.g. anxiety, depression, learning disorders) and non-psychiatric outcomes such as risky behaviours, accidents, and reduced life expectancy. A large-scale UK study found that adults with ADHD face a reduction in lifespan of up to 6–11 years, a disparity linked in part to comorbid health risks and underdiagnosis [9].

Functionally, ADHD impairs organisation, time management, emotional control, and sustained attention—areas critical to academic and occupational success. The neuroeconomic burden is significant, with direct and indirect costs reaching hundreds of billions of dollars globally [10].

5. Diagnostic and therapeutic advances

Diagnosis remains anchored in clinical criteria, based on behavioural symptomatology observed across settings. However, substantial heterogeneity and symptom overlap with other disorders (e.g. mood disorders, autism, learning disabilities) make accurate diagnosis challenging—particularly in adulthood and in female presentations [1].

Treatment has traditionally involved pharmacotherapy (stimulants such as methylphenidate or amphetamine; non-stimulants like atomoxetine or guanfacine) paired with psychotherapeutic and behavioural strategies. Recently, there has been growing interest in nonpharmacological interventions such as cognitive training, neurofeedback, mindfulness, exercise, and lifestyle modifications (e.g., sleep hygiene, diet, routine structured behaviour) [11].

The advent of technologies such as EEG-based deep learning models has opened new possibilities for objective and early diagnostics, particularly in school settings, such as the Siamese-based Convolutional Neural Network (CNN) model that achieved a high classification accuracy of 99.17% [12, 13].

6. Conclusion

This volume aims to synthesise and extend our understanding of ADHD by integrating foundational science with novel technological and interdisciplinary frameworks. Rather than presenting ADHD as a fixed disorder, we frame it as a dynamic, multifactorial condition with neurobiological, behavioural, developmental, and environmental dimensions. Understanding ADHD in its full complexity is essential not only for precise diagnosis and effective treatment but also for reducing stigma and enhancing life outcomes for those affected.

By embracing a multidisciplinary lens and engaging with innovations in neuroscience, chronobiology, AI-based diagnostics, and holistic care, we hope this book contributes to a more nuanced, compassionate, and impactful understanding of ADHD in the twenty-first century.

Author details

Marco Carotenuto
Child Neuropsychiatry, Department of Mental and Physical Health and Preventive Medicine, University of Campania "Luigi Vanvitelli", Caserta, Italy

*Address all correspondence to: marco.carotenuto@unicampania.it

References

[1] American Psychiatric Association. Diagnostic and Statistical Manual of Mental Disorders. DSM-5-TR. Arlington, Virginia: American Psychiatric Association Publishing; 2022. Disponibile su: https://psychiatryonline.org/doi/book/10.1176/appi.books.9780890425787

[2] Jurek L, Duchier A, Gauld C, Hénault L, Giroudon C, Fourneret P, et al. Sensory processing in individuals with attention-deficit/hyperactivity disorder compared with control populations: A systematic review and meta-analysis. Journal of the American Academy of Child and Adolescent Psychiatry. 2025;**S0890856725002096**:1-16

[3] Arrondo G, Solmi M, Dragioti E, Eudave L, Ruiz-Goikoetxea M, Ciaurriz-Larraz AM, et al. Associations between mental and physical conditions in children and adolescents: An umbrella review. Neuroscience and Biobehavioral Reviews. 2022;**137**:104662

[4] Grigore M, Ionică MV, Pătru L, Gheorman V, Wagner AP. Recent advances in the etiology and neural pathways underlying attention-deficit and hyperactivity disorder. Current Health Sciences Journal. 2025;**51**(1):14-25

[5] Bonvicini C, Cortese S, Maj C, Baune BT, Faraone SV, Scassellati C. DRD4 48 bp multiallelic variants as age-population-specific biomarkers in attention-deficit/hyperactivity disorder. Translational Psychiatry. 2020;**10**(1):70

[6] Carta A, Vainieri I, Rommel AS, Zuddas A, Kuntsi J, Sotgiu S, et al. Temperament dimensions and awakening cortisol levels in attention-deficit/hyperactivity disorder. Frontiers in Psychiatry. 2022;**13**:803001

[7] Cortese S. The neurobiology and genetics of attention-deficit/hyperactivity disorder (ADHD): What every clinician should know. The European Journal of Paediatric Neurology. 2012;**16**(5):422-433

[8] Hartman CA, Larsson H, Vos M, Bellato A, Libutzki B, Solberg BS, et al. Anxiety, mood, and substance use disorders in adult men and women with and without attention-deficit/hyperactivity disorder: A substantive and methodological overview. The European Journal of Paediatric Neurology. 2023;**151**:105209

[9] O'Nions E, El Baou C, John A, Lewer D, Mandy W, McKechnie DGJ, et al. Life expectancy and years of life lost for adults with diagnosed ADHD in the UK: Matched cohort study. British Journal of Psychiatry. 2025;**226**(5):261-268

[10] Li Y, Jönsson L. The health and economic burden of brain disorders: Consequences for investment in diagnosis, treatment, prevention and R&D. Cerebral Circulation - Cognition and Behavior. 2025;**8**:100377

[11] Cortese S, Moreno C. Advancing the evidence base for child and adolescent psychopharmacology. BMJ Mental Health. 2025;**28**(1):e301634

[12] Latifi B, Amini A, Motie NA. Siamese based deep neural network for ADHD detection using EEG signal. Computers in Biology and Medicine. 2024;**182**:109092

[13] Bansal J, Gangwar G, Aljaidi M, Alkoradees A, Singh G. EEG-based ADHD classification using autoencoder feature extraction and ResNet with double augmented attention mechanism. Brain Sciences. 2025;**15**(1):95

Chapter 2

ADHD in School Age Children: Overview

Fatimah Saeed Alahmari

Abstract

Attention Deficit Hyperactivity Disorder (ADHD), a prevalent neurodevelopmental disorder, significantly impacts millions of school-aged children globally through persistent inattention, hyperactivity, and impulsivity. This chapter synthesizes research on ADHD's profound effects on academic performance, social-emotional functioning, and daily life. The diagnostic process, involving clinical interviews, standardized rating scales, and differential diagnosis for comorbid conditions like anxiety and learning disorders, is detailed. Academic challenges stem from executive functioning deficits in working memory, time management, and organization, leading to difficulties in reading comprehension, mathematical errors, and lower standardized test scores. Long-term, students with ADHD face higher rates of grade repetition and high school dropout. Socially, impulsivity often results in peer conflict and social rejection. Emotionally, emotional dysregulation, characterized by frustration intolerance and low self-esteem, is common, exacerbated by high rates of anxiety and depression. The chapter advocates for evidence-based, multimodal interventions, including behavioral strategies (e.g., token economies, visual schedules), educational accommodations (e.g., IEPs/504 Plans, extended time, assistive technology), and pharmacological treatments (e.g., stimulants, non-stimulants). Emphasis is placed on collaboration *via* parent-teacher communication and advocacy through IDEA and Section 504 protections. Emerging trends like technology-based interventions (e.g., focus apps, and neurofeedback) and remote learning adaptations are also explored. By prioritizing early identification and individualized support, this chapter aims to empower stakeholders to foster resilience and success in children with ADHD.

Keywords: Attention Deficit Hyperactivity Disorder (ADHD), neurodevelopmental disorders, academic interventions, behavioral strategies, educational accommodations, pharmacological treatments, parent-teacher communication, comorbidity, emotional dysregulation, neurofeedback, remote learning

1. Introduction

Attention Deficit Hyperactivity Disorder (ADHD) is widely recognized as one of the most prevalent and extensively researched neurodevelopmental disorders impacting the pediatric population globally [1]. This intricate neurobiological condition is principally characterized by a pervasive and persistent pattern of inattention and/or hyperactivity-impulsivity that significantly interferes with an individual's functioning or development across multiple contexts, including academic, social, and occupational spheres [2]. While the exact etiology of ADHD remains multifaceted and is thought to involve a complex interplay of genetic, neurobiological, and environmental factors, its core symptoms typically emerge in early childhood, often before the age of 12, and can persist across the lifespan, influencing adolescence and adulthood, thereby necessitating a comprehensive understanding of its presentation and profound long-term implications [3].

Current epidemiological data consistently highlight the substantial prevalence of ADHD, with estimates suggesting it affects approximately 5–7.2% of school-aged children worldwide [4]. According to parent reports, 6.1 million American children aged 2–17 (9.4%) had ever been diagnosed with ADHD by a physician or other health care professional in 2016. Of them, 5.4 million had ADHD at the time of diagnosis, accounting for 8.4% of all children in the United States aged 2–17 and 89.4% of children who had ever received an ADHD diagnosis [5]. The enduring nature of ADHD, which frequently extends beyond childhood into adolescence and adulthood, further emphasizes the critical need for early and accurate diagnosis, alongside the implementation of sustained, evidence-based interventions to mitigate its potential adverse effects on an individual's developmental trajectory and overall quality of life [6].

Given the significant and multifaceted burden of this neurodevelopmental disorder on individual children, their families, and broader societal systems, a comprehensive and evidence-based approach to the identification, intervention, and ongoing advocacy for school-aged children with ADHD is paramount. This chapter aims to provide a detailed exposition of ADHD in this critical developmental period, synthesizing contemporary research findings from reputable medical journals and academic publications to elucidate the multifaceted impact of the disorder across academic, social, and emotional domains. Furthermore, it will meticulously delineate effective strategies for clinical management and educational support, emphasizing multimodal interventions that encompass behavioral strategies, educational accommodations, and, where clinically indicated and appropriate, pharmacological treatments. By fostering early identification, promoting individualized, strength-based support, and advocating for collaborative efforts among all key stakeholders—including educators, families, healthcare providers, and policymakers—this discourse seeks to empower children with ADHD, cultivate their inherent resilience, mitigate their challenges, and facilitate optimal developmental trajectories and long-term success. This holistic perspective is crucial for fostering an inclusive environment where children with ADHD can not only manage their symptoms but also thrive and reach their full potential.

2. Symptoms and diagnostic criteria

A precise understanding of the symptomatic presentation of ADHD is foundational for accurate diagnosis and effective intervention in school-aged children. The diagnostic criteria for ADHD are delineated in the Diagnostic and Statistical Manual of Mental Disorders, Fifth Edition (DSM-5) [7], which categorizes the disorder based on persistent patterns of inattention and/or hyperactivity-impulsivity that are developmentally inappropriate and significantly impair functioning across various contexts. These core symptom clusters are not merely transient behaviors but rather enduring characteristics that manifest across multiple settings, including home, school, and social environments [8].

DOI: http://dx.doi.org/10.5772/intechopen.1011335

2.1 Core symptoms

The hallmark features of ADHD are broadly classified into two primary symptom domains: inattention and hyperactivity-impulsivity. While these domains are distinct, they frequently co-occur and contribute synergistically to the functional impairments observed in affected children [2]. It is crucial to recognize that the manifestation of these symptoms must be considered in the context of the child's developmental stage, as behaviors such as high activity levels or occasional distractibility are normative in younger children. However, in ADHD, these behaviors are notably more severe, persistent, and disruptive than typically observed in age-matched peers [9].

2.1.1 Inattention

Inattention in the context of ADHD refers to a persistent difficulty in sustaining focus, maintaining vigilance, and resisting distracting stimuli, which significantly impedes a child's ability to engage effectively in tasks requiring sustained mental effort. This domain encompasses several distinct behavioral manifestations: Children with ADHD often struggle with sustained attention and vigilance during tasks, particularly those that are repetitive, lengthy, or perceived as uninteresting. This can manifest as a tendency to lose track of conversations, drift off during lectures, or become easily sidetracked when reading or working on assignments [2].

A characteristic feature of inattention is a propensity for making careless mistakes or overlooking details in academic work or other activities. This is often not due to a lack of understanding but rather a failure to meticulously attend to instructions or review work for accuracy. For instance, a child with ADHD might rush through a math problem, missing a crucial sign, or submit a written assignment riddled with superficial errors, despite possessing the requisite knowledge [9]. This can lead to a lower quality of academic output and diminished academic performance, even when the child has the intellectual capacity to succeed [10]. Children with inattention often exhibit significant forgetfulness in routine daily activities [1]. This can include misplacing essential items such as school books, homework assignments, or personal belongings; frequently forgetting to bring necessary materials to class; or failing to recall instructions given moments earlier [10].

2.1.2 Hyperactivity

Hyperactivity refers to excessive motor activity and restlessness that is often nonpurposeful and developmentally inappropriate for the child's age and context. This domain is characterized by an internal sense of restlessness that drives overt physical manifestations. Children demonstrating significant hyperactivity often exhibit a pervasive need for movement, even in settings where a calm demeanor is anticipated. This frequently presents as fidgeting with hands or feet, squirming in their seat, tapping objects, or constantly shifting their body position. This psychomotor agitation is commonly observed during structured activities such as classroom lessons, mealtimes, or quiet play, situations in which other children typically manage to remain still. A definitive characteristic of hyperactivity is the inability to remain seated in contexts where sitting is expected, like in a classroom, during dinner, or at formal gatherings. These children might frequently leave their seats, roam around the room, or stand up when their peers are seated. This is not merely a preference for being active, but an inherent struggle to inhibit motor impulses, which often leads to disruptions in structured environments and difficulties adhering to established rules. Additionally, hyperactive children may engage in excessive running, climbing, or other vigorous physical activities in inappropriate settings, such as indoors or in quiet public spaces. They may also display excessive verbal output, talking incessantly, blurting out answers, or making excessive noises, often without considering social cues or turn-taking protocols. This can significantly impede social interactions and further disrupt classroom settings, as their vocalizations might interfere with instruction or communication among peers [2].

2.1.3 Impulsivity

Impulsivity is defined by a tendency to act hastily without adequate forethought, a struggle to delay gratification, and significant challenges with response inhibition, reflecting a deficit in the ability to suppress immediate reactions or urges, often resulting in negative outcomes [11]. This manifests in several ways, including frequently interrupting others and exhibiting pronounced impatience, such as blurting out answers or intruding on activities, and struggling to wait their turn in various social scenarios, which can be perceived as rude. A critical facet of impulsivity is risky decision-making, where children engage in actions without considering potential negative consequences, such as taking physical risks or making rash comments. This lack of forethought and difficulty with delayed gratification can lead to dangerous situations and behavioral issues. Underlying these manifestations is a fundamental challenge with self-control, behavioral inhibition, and self-regulation; impulsive children often find it difficult to stop an ongoing behavior or regulate their emotional responses, leading to frequent outbursts and impacting their ability to follow rules and learn from mistakes [12].

2.2 DSM-5 subtypes

The Diagnostic and Statistical Manual of Mental Disorders, Fifth Edition (DSM-5), published by the American Psychiatric Association, serves as the authoritative guide for classifying mental disorders, including ADHD. The DSM-5 employs a categorical approach to ADHD diagnosis, recognizing the heterogeneity in its clinical presentation by classifying it into three distinct presentations, often referred to as "subtypes" in clinical practice. This classification is based on the predominant cluster of symptoms exhibited by an individual over the preceding 6 months, significantly impacting their functioning. Understanding these specific presentations is crucial for tailoring appropriate interventions and support for school-aged children [13].

2.2.1 Predominantly inattentive presentation (ADHD-PI)

The Predominantly Inattentive Presentation (ADHD-PI), formerly known as attention deficit disorder (ADD) without hyperactivity, is characterized by a prominent pattern of inattentive symptoms, with insufficient symptoms of hyperactivity-impulsivity to meet the criteria for those domains. For a diagnosis of ADHD-PI, an individual must exhibit six (or five for adolescents aged 17 and older and adults) or more symptoms of inattention. These symptoms are not merely occasional lapses in focus but are persistent, pervasive, and significantly impair functioning in academic, social, or occupational activities [14].

DOI: http://dx.doi.org/10.5772/intechopen.1011335

2.2.2 Predominantly Hyperactive-Impulsive Presentation (ADHD-HI)

The Predominantly Hyperactive-Impulsive Presentation (ADHD-HI) is diagnosed when an individual exhibits six (or five for adolescents aged 17 and older and adults) or more symptoms of hyperactivity-impulsivity, with insufficient symptoms of inattention to meet the criteria for that domain. This presentation is characterized by excessive motor activity and difficulties with impulse control that are significantly beyond what is developmentally expected for their age [15].

2.3 Diagnostic process

The accurate diagnosis of ADHD in school-aged children is a nuanced and comprehensive process that extends far beyond a single test or observation. It mandates a multi-informant, multi-method approach, integrating information from various sources and employing standardized assessment tools, all while carefully considering the developmental context of the child. Adherence to established clinical guidelines, such as those promulgated by the American Academy of Pediatrics (AAP) or the National Institute for Health and Care Excellence (NICE), is paramount to ensure diagnostic rigor and prevent misdiagnosis [16].

2.3.1 Clinical interviews

At the core of the diagnostic process are thorough clinical interviews. These interviews are systematically conducted with key informants who have sustained exposure to the child across different environments where symptoms might manifest.

2.3.2 Parent/caregiver interviews

Parent/caregiver interviews are crucial for diagnosing ADHD, providing a comprehensive developmental history. Key information gathered includes early childhood history regarding temperament, developmental milestones, and the emergence of hyperactive, impulsive, or inattentive behaviors from a young age. Clinicians also confirm symptom onset and duration, ensuring symptoms were present before age 12 and have persisted for at least 6 months, aligning with DSM-5 criteria [17].

2.3.3 Child interview

For school-aged children, an age-appropriate interview can provide valuable insight into their subjective experience of their symptoms, their self-perception, and their understanding of their difficulties. While younger children may offer limited self-report, older children and adolescents can often articulate their struggles with focus, restlessness, or impulsivity [18].

2.3.4 Teacher interviews/reports

Educators provide indispensable real-world data regarding the child's behavior and academic functioning within the structured demands of the school environment. Teachers can offer insights into attention span during lessons, adherence to classroom rules, social interactions with peers, and overall academic output, providing an external, objective perspective on symptom pervasiveness and severity [19].

2.4 Standardized rating scales

To quantify symptom severity and provide an objective comparison to normative data, standardized rating scales are indispensable tools in the diagnostic process. These scales are completed by parents, teachers, and, for older children, by the children themselves, ensuring a multi-informant perspective.

2.4.1 Conners 3rd edition (conners 3)

This is one of the most widely used and psychometrically sound rating scales for assessing ADHD and related problems in children and adolescents aged 6–18 years [20].

2.4.2 Other commonly used scales

In ADHD assessment, commonly used scales include the ADHD Rating Scale-5 (ADHD-RS-5), which directly measures the frequency and severity of both inattention and hyperactivity-impulsivity symptoms aligned with DSM-5 criteria. Additionally, the widely used Vanderbilt ADHD Diagnostic Parent and Teacher Rating Scales are freely available tools that provide DSM-5 symptom counts, impairment ratings, and screen for common comorbidities such as Oppositional Defiant Disorder (ODD), Conduct Disorder (CD), anxiety, and depression [21].

3. Comorbidities and differential diagnosis

A critical phase of the diagnostic process involves performing a thorough differential diagnosis to rule out other conditions that may mimic ADHD symptoms or to identify comorbidities (co-occurring conditions) that frequently accompany ADHD. Misattribution of symptoms to ADHD when another primary condition is present can lead to ineffective treatment [22]. **Table 1** highlights the common comorbidities in ADHD. **Table 1** summarizes differential diagnosis of ADHD comorbidities.

3.1 Anxiety disorders

Children with anxiety (e.g., Generalized Anxiety Disorder, Separation Anxiety Disorder) can present with inattention due to worry, intrusive thoughts, or

Condition	Overlap with ADHD	Distinguishing features	Recommended assessment tools
Anxiety Disorders	Restlessness, poor concentration	Worry precedes inattention	SCARED, MASC-2
Specific Learning Disorder	Academic underperformance	Skill deficits persist 1:1 instruction	WIAT-IV, Woodcock-Johnson
Autism Spectrum Disorder	Social difficulties	Stereotyped behaviors, sensory sensitivities	ADOS-2, SRS-2
Bipolar Disorder	Hyperactivity, impulsivity	Episodic mood elevation/irritability	K-SADS, YMRS

Table 1.
Differential diagnosis of ADHD comorbidities.

preoccupation, leading to difficulty concentrating. They might also exhibit restlessness or fidgeting, which can be mistaken for hyperactivity. A study by Elkins et al. [23] specifically examined inattention symptoms and the diagnosis of comorbid Attention-Deficit/Hyperactivity Disorder (ADHD) among youth with generalized anxiety disorder (GAD). Their findings suggest that while inattention can be a hallmark of both conditions, assessment tools for inattention may not always effectively distinguish between the two. The study highlights the importance of careful differential diagnosis, noting that a specific cutoff score on the Attention Problems Scale of the Child Behavior Checklist (CBCL) showed utility in identifying inattention specifically associated with ADHD among youth already diagnosed with GAD. This underscores the diagnostic challenge in differentiating anxiety-driven inattention from ADHD-related attentional deficits [23].

3.2 Mood disorders

Mood disorders can mimic ADHD symptoms, making differential diagnosis crucial. Depression in children can manifest as low mood, anhedonia (loss of pleasure), fatigue, and even psychomotor agitation, leading to apparent inattention, lack of motivation, or restlessness. Bipolar Disorder, though less common in prepubertal children, can present with a manic phase characterized by grandiosity, impulsivity, and increased energy, which may overlap significantly with core ADHD symptoms. A systematic review and meta-analysis by Sandstrom et al. [24] investigated the prevalence of ADHD in individuals with mood disorders, based on 92 studies including over 17,000 individuals. They found that the prevalence of ADHD in Bipolar Disorder is considerably high, ranging from 73% in childhood to 43% in adolescence, and 17% in adulthood. Similarly, for Major Depressive Disorder, the prevalence of ADHD was found to be 28% in childhood, 17% in adolescence, and 7% in adulthood. Notably, ADHD was three times more common in people with mood disorders compared to those without, and 1.7 times more common in bipolar disorder compared to Major Depressive Disorder. These findings underscore the significant comorbidity between ADHD and mood disorders, emphasizing the need for comprehensive assessment and treatment strategies that address both conditions [24].

3.3 Specific learning disorder (learning disabilities)

A child with a primary learning disability (e.g., dyslexia, dyscalculia) may become inattentive or disruptive specifically when faced with academically challenging tasks, but not necessarily in other domains. Comprehensive psychoeducational testing is often necessary to differentiate a primary learning disorder from ADHD, or to identify their co-occurrence, which is common [25].

3.4 Autism spectrum disorder (ASD)

There is significant overlap in symptoms between autism spectrum disorder (ASD) and Attention-Deficit/Hyperactivity Disorder (ADHD), particularly inattention and hyperactivity, and often in social communication difficulties. Differential diagnosis requires careful consideration of core ASD features like restricted interests, repetitive behaviors, and qualitative impairments in social interaction and communication. A study by Craig et al. [26] involving 181 subjects found that a group diagnosed with both ASD and ADHD exhibited a lower mean IQ level and higher autistic symptom severity compared to groups with only ASD or only ADHD. However, the ASD + ADHD group shared inattention and hyperactivity deficits, as well as some emotional and behavioral problems, with the ADHD group, while sharing adaptive behavior impairment with the ASD group. These findings emphasize the complex nature of this comorbidity and the need for a nuanced understanding of common and distinctive clinical features to inform accurate diagnosis and tailored interventions [26].

3.5 Impact on academic performance

ADHD exerts a profound and pervasive influence on the academic trajectory of school-aged children. Beyond the core symptoms of inattention and hyperactivity-impulsivity, a significant portion of this academic impairment can be attributed to underlying deficits in executive functions (EFs). Executive functions are a set of higher-order cognitive processes that enable goal-directed behavior, self-regulation, and adaptive responses to novel and complex situations. Indeed, a recent study by Español-Martín et al. [27] investigating 1287 Spanish students aged 5–17 has demonstrated that ADHD, alongside specific learning disorders, significantly impacts academic performance across both low-middle- and high-income populations, even when adjusted for comorbidity and other demographic factors. This highlights the pervasive nature of ADHD's influence on educational outcomes, underscoring the critical need for early detection and effective intervention strategies to improve academic functioning for these students [27].

3.6 Executive functioning deficits

Children with ADHD commonly struggle with specific facets of executive functioning, each contributing to a unique set of academic hurdles. These deficits are not merely manifestations of poor effort but reflect genuine neurocognitive differences that impact their ability to navigate the structured and demanding environment of school. A study by Schreiber et al. [28] utilized the NIH EXAMINER battery to assess executive function in children with ADHD, comparing them to typically developing controls. Their findings revealed that children with ADHD demonstrated significant impairments across various executive function domains, including working memory, inhibition, and set-shifting, even after controlling for age and IQ. This comprehensive assessment tool highlighted the pervasive nature of these deficits, providing further neurocognitive evidence for the executive function difficulties observed in children with ADHD [28].

3.7 Working memory

Working memory refers to the cognitive system responsible for temporarily holding and manipulating information in mind while performing complex cognitive tasks. It is a critical component of executive function, enabling individuals to keep multiple pieces of information active and accessible for immediate use. In children with ADHD, impairments in both verbal working memory (e.g., remembering a sequence of numbers or words) and visual-spatial working memory (e.g., recalling the location of objects or navigating a mental map) are commonly observed. A study by Kofler et al. [29] used a bifactor modeling approach to differentiate between working memory and short-term memory deficits in children with ADHD. Their findings indicated that while both working memory and short-term memory components are affected in ADHD, the deficits in working memory, particularly those related to the active manipulation of information, were more pronounced and contributed significantly to the overall cognitive profile of ADHD. This research provides a more nuanced understanding of the specific memory challenges faced by children with ADHD, moving beyond a simple distinction between verbal and visual-spatial impairments to highlight the core deficit in active information processing [29].

3.8 Time management

Time management, a complex executive function encompassing skills like planning, initiation, pacing, and progress monitoring, is often a distinct deficit for children with ADHD, who frequently struggle with an accurate sense of time. These difficulties significantly impair academic functioning, particularly in completing assignments on time. This pervasive issue stems from a combination of factors, including task initiation difficulties leading to procrastination, inaccurate time estimation where they consistently underestimate effort or overestimate available time, and challenges with pacing, resulting in uneven effort distribution and often last-minute rushing or incomplete work. As highlighted by Kreider et al. [30], who explored coping strategies for time-related and productivity challenges in young people with learning disabilities and ADHD, these struggles are deeply ingrained and require targeted interventions. Their work emphasizes that students with ADHD often face profound challenges in perceiving and managing time effectively, leading to significant academic and organizational difficulties, and suggests various strategies aimed at improving these crucial skills [30].

3.9 Organization

Organizational deficits profoundly affect children with ADHD, leading to academic hurdles. These children frequently misplace materials like textbooks and assignments, causing lost time and frustration. Forgetting deadlines is also common, as their difficulties hinder systematic tracking of tasks. Research by Bikic et al. [31] underscores the pervasive nature of these challenges and the importance of organizational skills training as a vital intervention. Further, LaCount et al. demonstrated that such training effectively improves academic performance in students with ADHD symptomatology, highlighting the significant impact of organizational skills on educational outcomes [32].

3.10 Classroom challenges: Reading, writing, and mathematics

Children with ADHD frequently encounter substantial challenges in reading and writing, fundamental literacy skills vital for academic advancement. These difficulties often stem from core symptoms of inattention and impulsivity, exacerbated by underlying executive function deficits. In reading, their comprehension is often reduced due to both internal (e.g., mind-wandering) and external (e.g., classroom noises) distractibility, which fragment their attention. Miller et al. [33] found that children with ADHD exhibit a "centrality deficit" in reading comprehension, showing their greatest impairment, relative to controls, in recalling central information from passages, even when word reading ability is controlled, and this difficulty is linked to deficits in working memory.

Writing presents significant hurdles as a complex executive function task, impacting their ability to produce written expression from ideation to final output, including poor planning, organization, and difficulty initiating tasks. Molitor et al. [34] found that adolescents with ADHD experience written expression impairment at rates similar to reading and mathematics impairment, with greater deficits observed in tasks requiring organization and attention to detail, especially in complex writing assignments. Soto et al. further clarified this, showing that underdeveloped working memory has significant direct effects on all three writing skills (written expression, spelling, and writing fluency) in children with ADHD, and also indirectly impacts written expression and spelling through ADHD symptoms, suggesting that underlying neurocognitive vulnerabilities are more involved in writing difficulties than overt behavioral symptoms [35].

3.11 Standardized testing

Standardized testing often disadvantages children with ADHD, leading to a disparity between their knowledge and performance, primarily due to time-management difficulties. The rigid, timed format of these assessments severely penalizes students with ADHD because of their challenges with time estimation, causing them to spend excessive time on difficult questions or rush through easier ones. Their pacing is also affected, making it hard to maintain a consistent and efficient rhythm throughout extended tests, which can lead to fatigue, waning focus, and consequently, incomplete sections or hurried, inaccurate responses. Despite possessing the necessary knowledge, many students with ADHD struggle with task completion, frequently failing to finish all questions within the allotted time, resorting to leaving answers blank or making rapid, incorrect guesses. Pritchard et al. [36] investigated the effectiveness of academic testing accommodations for students with ADHD. Their findings suggested that while extended time accommodations are frequently provided, their benefit on test scores can vary and might not fully bridge the gap in performance due to the complex interplay of ADHD symptoms and executive function deficits that impact test-taking behaviors beyond just time management. The study emphasizes the ongoing challenge of ensuring equitable assessment for students with ADHD and the need for a deeper understanding of how accommodations truly impact their performance [36].

3.12 Long-term academic outcomes

The academic challenges associated with ADHD in school-aged children are not merely transient difficulties but carry significant and persistent implications for their educational attainment and broader life trajectories. Without effective, sustained interventions, the functional impairments experienced in the classroom can accumulate, leading to severe educational disadvantages that profoundly impact an individual's future prospects. The long-term academic outcomes for students with ADHD underscore the critical imperative for early identification and comprehensive support [37].

3.13 Grade repetition

One of the most immediate and impactful long-term academic consequences for students with ADHD is a significantly elevated risk of grade repetition. Research consistently shows that children with ADHD are approximately three times more likely to repeat a grade than their neurotypical peers, with specific studies indicating that around 30–50% of children with ADHD will repeat at least one grade. This heightened risk stems from the core symptoms and executive functioning deficits of ADHD. A longitudinal study by Kent et al. [38] on male high school students with ADHD further highlighted this, finding that these students experienced substantial academic difficulties, including a significantly higher rate of grade retention compared to their non-ADHD peers. Their findings linked these academic struggles to persistent ADHD symptoms and associated deficits in areas like organization, time management, and academic effort, underscoring how these challenges directly contribute to the increased likelihood of grade repetition for students with ADHD [38].

4. Social and emotional implications

Beyond the significant academic hurdles, ADHD in school-aged children carries profound social and emotional implications that substantially impact their overall well-being and development. The core symptoms of inattention, hyperactivity, and impulsivity, along with associated executive functioning deficits, frequently interfere with a child's ability to navigate complex social interactions, regulate their emotions, and develop a positive self-concept. These challenges can lead to strained peer relationships, emotional dysregulation, and a heightened vulnerability to comorbid mental health conditions [39].

4.1 Peer relationships

The characteristic impulsivity and hyperactive behaviors of children with ADHD often create significant obstacles in forming and maintaining positive peer relationships. These behaviors can be perceived as disruptive, irritating, or intrusive by classmates, leading to social rejection and isolation. Research consistently indicates that children with ADHD are at a substantially higher risk of experiencing peer conflict. Specifically, a study by Licari [40] on the peer relations of children with ADHD found that approximately 50% of children with ADHD report experiencing peer conflict, underscoring the pervasive nature of these social difficulties within their daily interactions. This heightened rate of conflict can significantly impact their social development and overall well-being [40].

4.2 Emotional dysregulation

Emotional dysregulation refers to difficulties in managing and expressing emotions in socially appropriate and adaptive ways. This is a pervasive challenge for many children with ADHD, often considered a core feature of the disorder that significantly impacts their daily functioning. Children with ADHD frequently exhibit frustration intolerance, leading to disproportionate emotional reactions when faced with challenges, setbacks, or demands for sustained effort. Their difficulties with response inhibition, delayed gratification, and impaired executive functions mean they struggle to tolerate discomfort or persevere through difficult tasks. This chronic struggle in academic and social domains can severely erode a child's low self-esteem and self-worth, as they face a constant barrage of negative feedback from teachers regarding incomplete assignments, from parents about misbehavior, and from peers about social missteps [41].

5. Evidence-based interventions

Effective management of ADHD in school-aged children typically involves a multimodal approach, integrating a combination of evidence-based interventions tailored to the individual child's unique symptom profile, functional impairments, and co-occurring conditions. This comprehensive strategy aims to mitigate core ADHD symptoms, enhance adaptive skills, reduce associated impairments in academic and social domains, and improve overall quality of life. The most widely recognized and effective interventions fall broadly into behavioral strategies, educational accommodations, and pharmacological treatments. **Table 2** summarizes the evidence-based interventions for ADHD.

5.1 Behavioral strategies

Behavioral strategies serve as foundational interventions for ADHD, aiming to modify environmental factors to support desired behaviors and equip children and their families with adaptive coping skills. These strategies are often implemented consistently across various settings where the child faces difficulties. In the classroom, these methods, such as token economies and movement breaks, help students manage inattention, hyperactivity, and impulsivity, fostering a more conducive learning environment. As Pfiffner and Haack [43] emphasize, these classroom-based approaches are crucial for managing core ADHD symptoms and improving academic engagement. Home-based behavioral strategies are primarily delivered through Parent Training in Behavior Management (PTBM) or Parent Management Training (PMT). These programs empower parents by teaching them evidence-based behavioral principles like positive reinforcement, consistent consequences, and clear communication, often utilizing visual schedules to provide essential structure and predictability for the child. Pfiffner and Haack highlight the effectiveness of these parent-focused interventions in improving child behavior and reducing parental stress by equipping families with practical tools to manage ADHD symptoms in the home environment [43].

5.2 Pharmacological treatments

Pharmacological interventions for ADHD primarily involve two main classes of medication: stimulants and non-stimulants. **Table 3** compares stimulant vs. non-stimulant medications.

Intervention type	Examples	Mechanism	Key studies	Effect size
Behavioral	Token economy, visual schedules	Modifies environment to reinforce focus	Pfiffner and Haack [42]	Moderate (d = 0.6)
Pharmacological	Methylphenidate, atomoxetine	Enhances dopamine/norepinephrine	Brown et al. [42]	Large (d = 0.9)
Educational	IEPs, extended time	Reduces executive load	Pritchard et al. [36]	Moderate (d = 0.5)

Table 2.
Evidence-based interventions for ADHD.

Parameter	Methylphenidate (stimulant)	Atomoxetine (non-stimulant)
Onset of action	30–60 minutes	4–6 weeks
Duration	8–12 hours	24 hours
Common side effects	Reduced appetite, insomnia	Nausea, fatigue

Table 3.
Stimulant vs. non-stimulant medications.

5.2.1 Stimulants

Stimulants such as methylphenidate (e.g., Ritalin, Concerta) and amphetamines (e.g., Adderall, Vyvanse), work by increasing levels of dopamine and norepinephrine, particularly in the prefrontal cortex, which is crucial for executive functions like attention, impulse control, and planning. As reviewed by Brown et al. [42], these are considered the most effective pharmacological treatment for ADHD, with 70–80% of children experiencing significant symptom reduction within 30–60 minutes of administration. Their review further emphasizes that stimulants improve not only core ADHD symptoms but also associated impairments in academic performance, social functioning, and self-esteem, making them a cornerstone of ADHD management. They are available in various short-acting and long-acting formulations, allowing for individualized treatment plans [42].

5.2.2 Non-stimulants

Non-stimulants, including atomoxetine (Strattera), guanfacine extended-release (Intuniv), and clonidine extended-release (Kapvay), act through different neurochemical pathways. Atomoxetine is a selective norepinephrine reuptake inhibitor, while guanfacine and clonidine are alpha-2 adrenergic agonists that improve attention and reduce impulsivity/hyperactivity by acting on receptors in the prefrontal cortex. These serve as valuable alternatives for children who do not respond to stimulants, experience intolerable side effects, or have co-occurring conditions that stimulants might exacerbate. While generally less potent than stimulants, non-stimulants are still effective for many individuals, though their full therapeutic effect takes several weeks to manifest, as opposed to the rapid action of stimulants [44].

6. Case scenario (example)

6.1 Case study: Multimodal intervention in ADHD-C

Yousef, a 9-year-old with ADHD Combined Presentation (ADHD-C), exemplifies the interplay between pharmacological and behavioral interventions. Despite behavioral strategies (e.g., token economies at home) and classroom accommodations (e.g., preferential seating, extended time), his symptoms persisted: frequent off-task behavior, incomplete assignments, and impulsive interruptions.

Intervention: After ruling out comorbidities (e.g., anxiety, learning disorders), his pediatrician prescribed methylphenidate extended-release (a long-acting stimulant). Within 2 weeks, his teacher noted improved on-task behavior (sustained attention during 20-minute lessons) and reduced impulsivity (waiting his turn during group activities). These changes amplified the efficacy of existing behavioral supports—his responsiveness to visual reminders and token systems improved by 40%, per teacher reports.

6.2 Outcomes and considerations

Academic: Assignment completion rates rose from 30 to 75%, aligning with Soto et al.'s [35] findings on working memory improvements.

Social-Emotional: Peer conflicts decreased, and self-reported frustration during homework declined.

Challenges: Reduced midday appetite emerged, necessitating dietary adjustments (e.g., calorie-dense breakfasts).

This case underscores the synergy between stimulants and behavioral strategies [43], highlighting how medication can "prime" neurocognitive systems to engage with environmental supports. Regular follow-ups ensured dosage optimization and sustained adherence to IDEA-mandated accommodations.

7. Emerging research and innovations

The landscape of ADHD interventions is continuously evolving, driven by advancements in neuroscience, technology, and educational practices. Emerging research and innovative approaches offer new avenues for supporting school-aged children with ADHD, complementing traditional strategies and adapting to changing educational environments. These innovations often leverage technology to provide novel forms of support, from cognitive training to adaptive learning platforms. **Table 4** describes different types of multimodal intervention frameworks.

7.1 Technology-based interventions

The proliferation of digital tools and mobile applications has opened new frontiers for delivering interventions and supports for ADHD, often incorporating principles of gamification and personalized feedback. These interventions offer engaging and interactive ways to address core symptoms and executive function deficits. For instance, serious video games are being developed as therapeutic tools to treat ADHD, leveraging their interactive nature to train cognitive functions like attention

Domain	Strategies	Key outcomes (effect size)	Implementation tips
Behavioral	Token economy, self-monitoring	↑ Task completion	Combine home/school reinforcement
Pharmacological	Methylphenidate XR	↓ Core symptoms	Monitor growth and appetite
Educational	Extended time + graphic organizers	↑ Test scores	Train teachers in EF support
Technology	Neurofeedback apps	↑ Sustained attention	Limit session duration

Table 4.
Multimodal intervention framework.

and impulse control. As Sújar et al. [45] provide a tutorial guide for developing such games, they highlight the potential for these digital platforms to offer engaging and scalable treatment options. These technology-based approaches can provide immediate, tangible, and positive reinforcement, tapping into the brain's reward system and serving as nonintrusive reminders to stay on task, thus helping to mitigate impulsive behaviors or task switching. The ongoing development and evaluation of these digital interventions promise new avenues for personalized and accessible support for individuals with ADHD [45].

Neurofeedback, a noninvasive brain training technique and type of biofeedback, teaches individuals to self-regulate their brainwave activity in real-time. Electrodes placed on the scalp monitor brain electrical activity (EEG), and this information is presented to the individual through visual or auditory feedback, such as a video game that advances with desired brainwave patterns. As reviewed by Patil et al. [46], neurofeedback for children with ADHD aims to normalize brainwave patterns, specifically by increasing beta or sensorimotor rhythm (SMR) activity and decreasing theta activity, which are often dysregulated in individuals with ADHD. Their review highlights that this process helps children improve their ability to sustain attention, reduce impulsivity, and control hyperactivity by actively engaging with the feedback, thereby promoting better cognitive function through direct brain regulation [46].

7.2 Remote learning adaptations

The transition to remote and hybrid learning has necessitated specific adaptations to support students with ADHD, acknowledging both the unique challenges and potential advantages of virtual environments. While initial observations suggested increased difficulties for some ADHD students due to reduced structure and increased screen time, tailored strategies have proven beneficial. As highlighted by the European ADHD Guidelines Group, clinical experience during the COVID-19 pandemic underscored the critical need for specific considerations and adaptations when managing ADHD in remote contexts [47]. A critical adaptation is the implementation of structured online schedules. Students with ADHD benefit immensely from predictability and external structure, which compensate for challenges in executive functions like planning, organization, and time management. A clear, predictable timetable for synchronous instruction, asynchronous work, breaks, physical activity, and even nonacademic routines helps reduce cognitive load, minimize procrastination, and ensure academic demands are met without overwhelming the student. Providing these schedules in multiple formats, such as visual checklists or digital calendars with reminders, can further enhance their effectiveness. Indeed, research examining neurodivergent student experiences, including those with ADHD, in higher education emphasizes that such structured support is fundamental for improving their access and inclusion within educational environments [48].

8. Conclusion

ADHD represents a complex neurodevelopmental condition that profoundly impacts school-aged children across multiple facets of their lives. As explored throughout this chapter, the core symptoms of inattention, hyperactivity, and impulsivity are not merely behavioral quirks but manifest as significant impairments in academic performance, social interactions, and emotional well-being. These challenges, if unaddressed, can lead to serious long-term consequences, including increased rates of grade repetition and high school dropout.

The pervasive nature of ADHD necessitates a comprehensive and nuanced understanding of its impact. In the classroom, difficulties with sustained attention translate into reduced reading comprehension and careless errors in mathematics. Time-management deficits often undermine performance on standardized tests, potentially misrepresenting a student's true capabilities. Beyond academics, the impulsive behaviors characteristic of ADHD frequently leads to social rejection and peer conflict, contributing to feelings of isolation. Internally, children with ADHD often grapple with emotional dysregulation, marked by frustration intolerance and low self-esteem, which are compounded by chronic academic and social struggles. The high prevalence of comorbid conditions like anxiety and depression further underscores the intricate psychological landscape faced by these children, demanding a holistic view for effective support.

In conclusion, while ADHD presents significant challenges for school-aged children, it is a highly treatable condition. With early diagnosis, individualized multimodal interventions, dedicated collaboration among all stakeholders, and informed advocacy, children with ADHD can overcome substantial barriers, harness their strengths, and ultimately thrive academically, socially, and emotionally, realizing their full potential. Continued commitment to research, compassionate practice, and strong advocacy remains essential to ensure every child with ADHD has the opportunity to succeed.

Acknowledgements

I extend my deepest gratitude to the individuals and institutions whose expertise, support, and collaboration made this chapter possible.

Conflict of interest

The author declares no known conflicts of interest, financial or otherwise, that could influence the content, interpretation, or recommendations presented in this chapter. No funding was received from pharmaceutical companies, educational technology firms, or other entities with a commercial stake in ADHD treatments or interventions discussed herein.

Appendices and nomenclature

ADHD	Attention Deficit Hyperactivity Disorder—a neurodevelopmental disorder characterized by persistent patterns of inattention and/or hyperactivity-impulsivity.
ADHD-C	combined presentation of ADHD—a diagnostic subtype where criteria for both inattention and hyperactivity-impulsivity are met.

ADHD-HI	Predominantly Hyperactive-Impulsive Presentation of ADHD—a diagnostic subtype where criteria for hyperactivity-impulsivity are met, but not for inattention.
ADHD-PI	Predominantly Inattentive Presentation of ADHD—a diagnos tic subtype where criteria for inattention are met, but not for hyperactivity-impulsivity.
AAP	American Academy of Pediatrics—a professional organization of pediatricians in the United States.
Assistive Technology	any item, piece of equipment, or product system, whether acquired commercially off the shelf, modified, or customized, that is used to increase, maintain, or improve functional capabilities of individuals with disabilities.
Comorbidity	the presence of two or more distinct medical or psychiatric conditions occurring simultaneously in an individual.
DSM-5	Diagnostic and Statistical Manual of Mental Disorders, Fifth Edition—the standard classification of mental disorders used by mental health professionals in the United States.
Emotional Dysregulation	difficulties in managing and expressing emotions in socially appropriate and adaptive ways.
Executive Functions (EFs)	A set of higher-order cognitive processes that enable goal-directed behavior, self-regulation, and adaptive responses, including working memory, planning, organization, and impulse control.
FAPE	Free Appropriate Public Education—a legal right guaranteed by IDEA, ensuring special education and related services are provided at public expense.
Frustration Intolerance	a low threshold for enduring frustration, leading to disproportionate emotional reactions when faced with challenges or setbacks.
Hyperactivity	excessive motor activity and restlessness that is often non-purposeful and developmentally inappropriate.
IDEA	Individuals with Disabilities Education Act—a federal law that ensures children with disabilities receive a free appropriate public education.

IEP	Individualized Education Program—a legally binding document under IDEA that outlines specialized instruction and services for eligible students.
Impulsivity	a tendency to act hastily without forethought, difficulty in delaying gratification, and challenges with response inhibition.
Inattention	persistent difficulty in sustaining focus, maintaining vigilance, and cresisting distracting stimuli.
Least Restrictive Environment (LRE)	a principle under IDEA that mandates children with disabilities be educated with non-disabled children to the maximum extent appropriate.
Multimodal Approach	acomprehensive treatment strategy that integrates multiple evidence-based interventions (e.g., behavioral, educational, pharmacological).
Neurodevelopmental Disorder	a group of conditions with onset in the developmental period, characterized by developmental deficits that produce impairments of personal, social, academic, or occupational functioning.
Neurofeedback	a non-invasive brain training technique that teaches individuals to self-regulate their brainwave activity in real-time.
NICE	National Institute for Health and Care Excellence—a public body in the UK that provides national guidance and advice to improve health and social care.
OHI	Other Health Impairment—a disability category under IDEA that may include ADHD if it significantly impacts a child's strength, vitality, or alertness, affecting educational performance.
Organization	the executive function involving the ability to create and maintain order in physical space, information, and tasks.
Parent Management Training (PMT)	an evidence-based behavioral intervention that teaches parents skills to manage their child's challenging behaviors.
Section 504	Section 504 of the Rehabilitation Act of 1973—a civil rights law that prohibits discrimination against individuals with disabilities and ensures accommodations for equal access to education.
Stimulants	a class of pharmacological treatments (e.g., methylphenidate, amphetamines) commonly used for ADHD, which increase

	dopamine and norepinephrine levels in the brain.
Time Management	the executive function involving the ability to perceive, estimate, allocate, and regulate time effectively to achieve goals and complete tasks.
Working Memory	the cognitive system responsible for temporarily holding and manipulating information in mind while performing complex cognitive tasks.

Author details

Fatimah Saeed Alahmari[1,2]

1 Developmental and Behavioural Pediatrics Specialized Clinics, Eradah and Mental Health Complex, Third Health Cluster, Riyadh, Saudi Arabia

2 College of Medicine, Alfaisal University, Saudi Arabia

*Address all correspondence to: fatimahsa@hotmail.com

References

[1] Singh A, Yeh CJ, Verma N, Das AK. Overview of attention deficit hyperactivity disorder in young children. Health Psychology Research. 2015;**3**(2):2115. DOI: 10.4081/hpr.2015.2115

[2] Magnus W, Anilkumar AC, Shaban K. Attention deficit hyperactivity disorder. In: StatPearls. Treasure Island (FL): StatPearls Publishing; 2025. Available from: https://www.ncbi.nlm.nih.gov/books/NBK441838/

[3] Núñez-Jaramillo L, Herrera-Solís A, Herrera-Morales WV. ADHD: Reviewing the causes and evaluating solutions. Journal of Personalized Medicine. 2021;**11**(3):166. DOI: 10.3390/jpm11030166

[4] Abdelnour E, Jansen MO, Gold JA. ADHD diagnostic trends: Increased recognition or overdiagnosis? Missouri Medicine. 2022;**119**(5):467-473

[5] Danielson ML, Bitsko RH, Ghandour RM, Holbrook JR, Kogan MD, Blumberg SJ. Prevalence of parent-reported ADHD diagnosis and associated treatment among U.S. children and adolescents, 2016. Journal of Clinical Child and Adolescent Psychology. 2018;**47**(2):199-212. DOI: 10.1080/15374416.2017.1417860 Epub 2018 Jan 24

[6] Hinshaw SP, Arnold LE. For the MTA cooperative group. ADHD, multimodal treatment, and longitudinal outcome: Evidence, paradox, and challenge. Wiley Interdisciplinary Reviews: Cognitive Science. 2015;**6**(1):39-52. DOI: 10.1002/wcs.1324

[7] Substance Abuse and Mental Health Services Administration. DSM-5 Changes: Implications for Child Serious Emotional Disturbance. Rockville (MD): Substance Abuse and Mental Health Services Administration (US); 2016. Table 7, DSM-IV to DSM-5 Attention-Deficit/Hyperactivity Disorder Comparison. Available from: https://www.ncbi.nlm.nih.gov/books/NBK519712/table/ch3.t3/

[8] Cabral MDI, Liu S, Soares N. Attention-deficit/hyperactivity disorder: Diagnostic criteria, epidemiology, risk factors and evaluation in youth. Translational Pediatrics. 2020;**9** (Suppl. 1):S104-S113. DOI: 10.21037/tp.2019.09.08

[9] Musullulu H. Evaluating attention deficit and hyperactivity disorder (ADHD): A review of current methods and issues. Frontiers in Psychology. 2025;**16**:1466088. DOI: 10.3389/fpsyg.2025.1466088

[10] Gawrilow C, Kühnhausen J, Schmid J, Stadler G. Hyperactivity and motoric activity in ADHD: Characterization, assessment, and intervention. Frontiers in Psychiatry. 2014;**5**:171. DOI: 10.3389/fpsyt.2014.00171

[11] Barrett ES, Stanford MS. Impulsiveness. In: Costello CG, editor. Personality Characteristics of the Personality Disordered. New York: Wiley; 1996. pp. 91-119

[12] Winstanley CA, Eagle DM, Robbins TW. Behavioral models of impulsivity in relation to ADHD: Translation between clinical and preclinical studies. Clinical Psychology Review. 2006;**26**(4):379-395. DOI: 10.1016/j.cpr.2006.01.001. Epub 2006 Feb 28

[13] Regier DA, Kuhl EA, Kupfer DJ. The DSM-5: Classification and criteria changes. World Psychiatry.

2013;**12**(2):92-98. DOI: 10.1002/wps.20050

[14] de la Peña IC, Pan MC, Thai CG, Alisso T. Attention-deficit/hyperactivity disorder predominantly inattentive subtype/presentation: Research progress and translational studies. Brain Sciences. 2020;**10**(5):292. DOI: 10.3390/brainsci10050292

[15] Gibbins C, Weiss MD, Goodman DW, Hodgkins PS, Landgraf JM, Faraone SV. ADHD-hyperactive/impulsive subtype in adults. Mental Illness. 2010;**2**(1):e9. DOI: 10.4081/mi.2010.e9

[16] Wolraich ML, Hagan JF Jr, Allan C, Chan E, Davison D, Earls M, et al. Clinical practice guideline for the diagnosis, evaluation, and treatment of attention-deficit/hyperactivity disorder in children and adolescents. Pediatrics. 2019;**144**(4):e20192528. DOI: 10.1542/peds.2019-2528. Erratum in: Pediatrics. 2020 Mar;145(3):e20193997. doi: 10.1542/peds.2019-3997

[17] De Los Reyes A, Augenstein TM, Wang M, Thomas SA, Drabick DAG, Burgers DE, et al. The validity of the multi-informant approach to assessing child and adolescent mental health. Psychological Bulletin. 2015;**141**(4):858-900. DOI: 10.1037/a0038498. Epub 2015 Apr 27

[18] Slobodin O, Davidovitch M. Primary school children's self-reports of attention deficit hyperactivity disorder-related symptoms and their associations with subjective and objective measures of attention deficit hyperactivity disorder. Frontiers in Human Neuroscience. 2022;**16**:806047. DOI: 10.3389/fnhum.2022.806047

[19] Aldabbagh R, Daley D, Sayal K, Glazebrook C. Exploring the unmet needs of teachers of young children with ADHD symptoms: A qualitative study. Children (Basel). 2024;**11**(9):1053. DOI: 10.3390/children11091053

[20] Izzo VA, Donati MA, Novello F, Maschietto D, Primi C. The Conners 3-short forms: Evaluating the adequacy of brief versions to assess ADHD symptoms and related problems. Clinical Child Psychology and Psychiatry. 2019;**24**(4):791-808. DOI: 10.1177/1359104519846602. Epub 2019 May 10

[21] Nasser A, Kosheleff AR, Hull JT, Liranso T, Qin P, Busse GD, et al. Translating attention-deficit/hyperactivity disorder rating scale-5 and weiss functional impairment rating scale-parent effectiveness scores into clinical global impressions clinical significance levels in four randomized clinical trials of SPN-812 (Viloxazine Extended-Release) in children and adolescents with attention-deficit/hyperactivity disorder. Journal of Child and Adolescent Psychopharmacology. 2021;**31**(3):214-226. DOI: 10.1089/cap.2020.0148. Epub 2021 Feb 17

[22] Gnanavel S, Sharma P, Kaushal P, Hussain S. Attention deficit hyperactivity disorder and comorbidity: A review of literature. World Journal of Clinical Cases. 2019;**7**(17):2420-2426. DOI: 10.12998/wjcc.v7.i17.2420

[23] Elkins RM, Carpenter AL, Pincus DB, Comer JS. Inattention symptoms and the diagnosis of comorbid attention-deficit/hyperactivity disorder among youth with generalized anxiety disorder. Journal of Anxiety Disorders. 2014;**28**(8):754-760. DOI: 10.1016/j.janxdis.2014.09.003. Epub 2014 Sep 17

[24] Sandstrom A, Perroud N, Alda M, Uher R, Pavlova B. Prevalence of attention-deficit/hyperactivity disorder

in people with mood disorders: A systematic review and meta-analysis. Acta Psychiatrica Scandinavica. 2021;**143**(5):380-391. DOI: 10.1111/acps.13283. Epub 2021 Feb 15

[25] Verma N, Pawar KD, Shah HR, Shelke SB. SLD with and without ADHD: Comparison of cognitive profiles. Industrial Psychiatry Journal. 2023;**32**(2):448-451. DOI: 10.4103/ipj.ipj_6_23. Epub 2023 Aug 11

[26] Craig F, Lamanna AL, Margari F, Matera E, Simone M, Margari L. Overlap between autism spectrum disorders and attention deficit hyperactivity disorder: Searching for distinctive/common clinical features. Autism Research. 2015;**8**(3):328-337. DOI: 10.1002/aur.1449. Epub 2015 Jan 20

[27] Español-Martín G, Pagerols M, Prat R, Rivas C, Ramos-Quiroga JA, Casas M, et al. The impact of attention-deficit/hyperactivity disorder and specific learning disorders on academic performance in Spanish children from a low-middle- and a high-income population. Frontiers in Psychiatry. 2023;**14**:1136994. DOI: 10.3389/fpsyt.2023.1136994

[28] Schreiber JE, Possin KL, Girard JM, Rey-Casserly C. Executive function in children with attention deficit/hyperactivity disorder: The NIH EXAMINER battery. Journal of the International Neuropsychological Society. 2014;**20**(1):41-51. DOI: 10.1017/S1355617713001100. Epub 2013 Oct 8

[29] Kofler MJ, Singh LJ, Soto EF, Chan ESM, Miller CE, Harmon SL, et al. Working memory and short-term memory deficits in ADHD: A bifactor modeling approach. Neuropsychology. 2020;**34**(6):686-698. DOI: 10.1037/neu0000641. Epub 2020 May 21

[30] Kreider CM, Medina S, Slamka MR. Strategies for coping with time-related and productivity challenges of young people with learning disabilities and attention-deficit/hyperactivity disorder. Children (Basel). 2019;**6**(2):28. DOI: 10.3390/children6020028

[31] Bikic A, Dalsgaard S, Olsen KD, Sukhodolsky DG. Organizational skills training for children with ADHD: Study protocol for a randomized, controlled trial. Trials. 2021;**22**(1):752. DOI: 10.1186/s13063-021-05499-9

[32] LaCount PA, Hartung CM, Shelton CR, Stevens AE. Efficacy of an organizational skills intervention for college students with ADHD symptomatology and academic difficulties. Journal of Attention Disorders. 2018;**22**(4):356-367. DOI: 10.1177/1087054715594423. Epub 2015 Aug 7

[33] Miller AC, Keenan JM, Betjemann RS, Willcutt EG, Pennington BF, Olson RK. Reading comprehension in children with ADHD: Cognitive underpinnings of the centrality deficit. Journal of Abnormal Child Psychology. 2013;**41**(3):473-483. DOI: 10.1007/s10802-012-9686-8

[34] Molitor SJ, Langberg JM, Evans SW. The written expression abilities of adolescents with attention-deficit/hyperactivity disorder. Research in Developmental Disabilities. 2016;**51-52**:49-59. DOI: 10.1016/j.ridd.2016.01.005. Epub 2016 Jan 21

[35] Soto EF, Irwin LN, Chan ESM, Spiegel JA, Kofler MJ. Executive functions and writing skills in children with and without ADHD. Neuropsychology. 2021;**35**(8):792-808. DOI: 10.1037/neu0000769. Epub 2021 Sep 27

[36] Pritchard AE, Koriakin T, Carey L, Bellows A, Jacobson L, Mahone EM.

Academic testing accommodations for ADHD: Do they help? Learning Disabilities (Pittsburgh, PA.). 2016;**21**(2):67-78. DOI: 10.18666/LDMJ-2016-V21-I2-7414

[37] Loe IM, Feldman HM. Academic and educational outcomes of children with ADHD. Journal of Pediatric Psychology. 2007;**32**(6):643-654. DOI: 10.1093/jpepsy/jsl054

[38] Kent KM, Pelham WE Jr, Molina BS, Sibley MH, Waschbusch DA, Yu J, et al. The academic experience of male high school students with ADHD. Journal of Abnormal Child Psychology. 2011;**39**(3):451-462. DOI: 10.1007/s10802-010-9472-4

[39] Classi P, Milton D, Ward S, Sarsour K, Johnston J. Social and emotional difficulties in children with ADHD and the impact on school attendance and healthcare utilization. Child and Adolescent Psychiatry and Mental Health. 2012;**6**(1):33. DOI: 10.1186/1753-2000-6-33

[40] Licari JE. Peer relations of children with attention deficit hyperactivity disorder. 1997. p. 89. Graduate Research Papers. 1108. Available from: https://scholarworks.uni.edu/grp/1108

[41] Shaw P, Stringaris A, Nigg J, Leibenluft E. Emotion dysregulation in attention deficit hyperactivity disorder. The American Journal of Psychiatry. 2014;**171**(3):276-293. DOI: 10.1176/appi.ajp.2013.13070966

[42] Brown KA, Samuel S, Patel DR. Pharmacologic management of attention deficit hyperactivity disorder in children and adolescents: A review for practitioners. Translational Pediatrics. 2018;**7**(1):36-47. DOI: 10.21037/tp.2017.08.02

[43] Pfiffner LJ, Haack LM. Behavior management for school-aged children with ADHD. Child and Adolescent Psychiatric Clinics of North America. 2014;**23**(4):731-746. DOI: 10.1016/j.chc.2014.05.014. Epub 2014 Aug 10

[44] Vilus JT, Engelhard C. Nonstimulant medications for treatment of attention-deficit/hyperactivity disorder in children and adolescents. Pediatric Annals. 2025;**54**(1):e27-e33. DOI: 10.3928/19382359-20241007-07, Epub 2025 Jan 1

[45] Sújar A, Martín-Moratinos M, Rodrigo-Yanguas M, Bella-Fernández M, González-Tardón C, Delgado-Gómez D, et al. Developing serious video games to treat attention deficit hyperactivity disorder: Tutorial guide. JMIR Serious Games. 2022;**10**(3):e33884. DOI: 10.2196/33884

[46] Patil AU, Madathil D, Fan Y-T, Tzeng OJL, Huang C-M, Huang H-W. Neurofeedback for the education of children with ADHD and specific learning disorders: A review. Brain Sciences. 2022;**12**:1238. DOI: 10.3390/brainsci12091238

[47] Santosh P, Cortese S, Hollis C, Bölte S, Daley D, Coghill D, et al. Remote assessment of ADHD in children and adolescents: Recommendations from the European ADHD Guidelines Group following the clinical experience during the COVID-19 pandemic. European Child & Adolescent Psychiatry. 2023;**32**(6):921-935. DOI: 10.1007/s00787-023-02148-1. Epub 2023 Feb 11

[48] Butcher L, Lane S. Neurodivergent (autism and ADHD) student experiences of access and inclusion in higher education: An ecological systems theory perspective. Higher Education. 2024. DOI: 10.1007/s10734-024-01319-6

Chapter 3

Perspective Chapter: The Impact of Circadian Rhythm Dysregulation in the Treatment Resistance and Medication Efficacy of ADHD across the Lifespan

Alessandra Carta, Vanna Cavassa and Stefano Sotgiu

Abstract

This work explores how circadian rhythm dysregulation (*CRD*) affects individuals with Attention-Deficit/Hyperactivity Disorder (*ADHD*), focusing on its impact on *comorbidities, treatment resistance*, and the *effectiveness* of medications from early childhood through young adulthood. ADHD is increasingly understood not only as a neurodevelopmental condition but also as one often marked by *misalignment* of internal circadian rhythms. This misalignment contributes to *sleep disturbances*, which in turn can *aggravate core symptoms* such as inattention, impulsivity, emotional dysregulation, and executive dysfunction. CRD *interferes with treatment* in several ways. The circadian system influences *how* medications are *absorbed* and *metabolized*, meaning that individuals with disrupted rhythms may experience *reduced efficacy* or *stronger side effects* depending on the timing of administration. Sleep deprivation and altered melatonin cycles can further limit the benefits of stimulant treatments. ADHD frequently *coexists* with sleep and mood disorders, as well as metabolic disturbances, which make *treatment more complex* and call for individualized care. The effects of circadian disruption also *change over the course of development*: in early childhood, it can intensify hyperactivity; in school-age children, it can impair learning and attention; in adolescents, phase delays and poor sleep hygiene complicate medication timing; and in young adults, irregular routines often worsen circadian misalignment and treatment response. *Addressing CRD* is therefore *essential* for *improving clinical outcomes*. Interventions such as light therapy, melatonin supplementation, sleep-focused behavioral strategies, and timing medications in line with circadian patterns offer promising avenues for more effective, personalized ADHD treatment.

Keywords: ADHD across lifespan, circadian rhythm dysregulation, medication efficacy, treatment resistance, sleep and other comorbidities of ADHD

1. Introduction

Disruptions in circadian rhythm are strongly associated with *several psychiatric disorders*, including *major depressive disorder*, *bipolar disorder*, and *schizophrenia* [1, 2].

In fact, circadian disturbances are included among the diagnostic criteria for these conditions. Such dysregulations are also closely linked to *sleep disorders*, including *insomnia* and *fragmented sleep* [3]. Alterations in the circadian system may help explain the *frequent co-occurrence of sleep and psychiatric disorders* and are increasingly being explored as potential *therapeutic targets* [4].

Circadian dysregulation has also been implicated in attention-deficit/hyperactivity disorder (*ADHD*), which frequently coexists with other *psychiatric and neurodevelopmental conditions*, complicating both *diagnosis* and *treatment* [5]. Common comorbidities include oppositional defiant disorder, conduct disorder, anxiety and mood disorders, autism spectrum disorder, specific learning disorders, and sleep disturbances [6].

Recent research underscores the *heterogeneity of ADHD*, advocating for a *dimensional rather* than a purely categorical conceptualization. This approach acknowledges a *continuum* of symptom severity and diagnostic overlap, potentially *improving clinical assessment* and enabling more *personalized treatment* strategies [7].

To understand how circadian disruption affects individuals with ADHD, it is first necessary to outline how the circadian system functions at physiological and molecular levels.

1.1 Circadian rhythm

The sleep-wake cycle is regulated by two main processes: the *homeostatic process* (Process S) and the *circadian process* (Process C). The circadian rhythm is an internal biological timing system that aligns with the natural alternation of light and dark in the environment. This rhythm is primarily controlled by the *suprachiasmatic nucleus (SCN)*, a small cluster of neurons in the *hypothalamus* that functions as the body's central clock. In humans, this internal rhythm generally spans about 24 hours [5, 8].

Process S is a homeostatic mechanism that reflects sleep pressure: the longer an individual remains awake, the greater the physiological drive for sleep. *Process C*, by contrast, is a circadian mechanism that modulates the sensitivity to sleep pressure. It is regulated by internal biological signals, including fluctuations in cortisol levels and core body temperature [9, 10].

The SCN receives light-based input that helps it stay in sync with the external environment [11, 12]. This regulation happens through three main pathways. The first is the *retinohypothalamic tract*, which directly sends light information from specialized retinal cells to the SCN. The second is the *geniculohypothalamic tract*, which transmits signals indirectly from the lateral geniculate nucleus. A third source comes from the *raphe nuclei*, which send serotonergic signals that contribute to fine-tuning the clock based on factors beyond light, such as behavior or physical activity [13, 14].

A key downstream pathway involves the *superior cervical ganglia*, which transmit signals to the *pineal gland*, *via* GABAergic pathways, regulating the circadian release of *melatonin*, which is synthesized in the pinealocytes from the precursor tryptophan. The secretion of melatonin exhibits a clear circadian rhythm, with peak plasma levels usually between 02:00 and 03:00 am [15].

On a molecular level, our circadian rhythms are driven by a set of genes that follow a rhythmic cycle of activation and inhibition. A set of core clock genes, including *CLOCK*, *BMAL1*, *PER*, *CRY*, *REV-ERBα*, and *RORA*, work together in feedback loops to keep time within our cells [16]. Beyond these loops, various chemical modifications affect how stable these proteins are, subtly adjusting the pace of the cycle. Notably, these clock genes do not just keep track of time, they also influence a wide range of other biological processes. Research shows that nearly *half of all protein-coding genes* in the body show circadian patterns of activity in at least one tissue [17].

Cortisol, the main glucocorticoid produced by the adrenal glands, plays a central role in the hypothalamic-pituitary-adrenal (HPA) axis and also acts as a key hormonal output of the circadian system. Its secretion is regulated by the SCN through downstream pathways involving *arginine vasopressin* and *corticotropin-releasing hormone*. Cortisol follows a well-defined circadian pattern: levels rise in the early morning, peaking shortly after awakening, and gradually decline throughout the day. Exposure to light upon waking has been shown to enhance this morning peak. Beyond its role in stress response, cortisol also contributes to the *entrainment of peripheral circadian oscillators*, helping to synchronize internal rhythms across tissues [18].

2. Circadian dysregulation and its relevance in ADHD

2.1 Pathophysiological mechanism

Over the years, *circadian rhythm alterations* in ADHD have been increasingly investigated as researchers attempt to find the unique factors which may distinguish people with this condition from those without. A key question is whether circadian perturbation is a *causal factor* for ADHD or if it is a *downstream phenomenon* of ADHD symptomatology [19, 20].

Literature reports that individuals with ADHD are more likely to have a preference for *eveningness*, a chronotype characterized by a later sleep and waking up [21]. This pattern has been associated with an exacerbation of core symptoms of ADHD, even in general populations, such as inattention, impulsivity, risk-taking, novelty, and sensation seeking, and difficulties in executive and mnemonic functioning [22, 23].

Another commonly observed circadian phenotype in this population is *delayed sleep phase syndrome (DSPS)*, where the time of onset of sleep occurs significantly later than in typical development [24]. These findings are further corroborated by both subjective measures like *Morningness–Eveningness Questionnaire (MEQ)* and the *Munich Chronotype Questionnaire (MCTQ)*, as well as objective measures like *actigraphy* [25].

Alterations in melatonin signaling have drawn considerable interest in the study of circadian rhythm dysfunction in ADHD. One recurring observation is a *delayed dim light melatonin onset (DLMO)*, which points to a broader delay in the circadian phase. This shift appears particularly relevant in individuals with *comorbid sleep-onset insomnia* or *delayed sleep phase disorder* (DSPD), though it also shows up in adults with chronic difficulties falling asleep [26].

However, while the *timing of melatonin secretion* is consistently found to be delayed, the findings regarding *absolute melatonin levels* are less consistent. Several studies using *salivary samples* have reported *no significant differences* in melatonin concentrations between ADHD subjects and controls [27]. In contrast, studies assessing *urinary melatonin metabolites*, such as 6-hydroxymelatonin sulfate (6-OH-MS) or 6-sulfatoxymelatonin, have found *elevated excretion* in children and adolescents with ADHD, regardless of the time of day [28, 29]. This apparent discrepancy has led to speculation that the metabolism of melatonin in ADHD may be altered, possibly involving a *faster catabolism or breakdown of the hormone*. As a result, individuals with ADHD might experience a narrower temporal window in which melatonin concentrations are elevated, potentially reducing the hormone's effectiveness in promoting sleep onset [27, 29].

Another hypothesis is that this change in melatonin metabolism may be a consequence of *frequent sleep disruptions* or other underlying neurophysiological abnormalities, such as an increase in *paroxysmal EEG activity*, which are more prevalent in children with ADHD [28]. Some authors speculate the increased production and rapid clearance of melatonin could reflect compensatory mechanisms in the setting of chronic circadian misalignment and/or sleep fragmentation [29].

Melatonin and cortisol are both regulated by the *central circadian pacemaker* in the SCN; for this reason, alterations in one hormone often imply *broader circadian dysfunction* [6].

In this context, *cortisol* has been investigated as a marker for the modulation of arousal in ADHD, including the awakening response.

Cortisol has also been examined in relation to *arousal regulation* in ADHD. Produced by the adrenal glands *via* the hypothalamic-pituitary-adrenal (*HPA*) axis, cortisol follows a well-known circadian rhythm. It typically peaks shortly after waking—this is referred to as the *cortisol awakening response (CAR)*—and then *gradually declines* throughout the day [30, 31]. In individuals with ADHD, several studies have suggested that this rhythm may be *disrupted* [32, 33].

For instance, metaanalytic findings report that children with ADHD, whether medicated or not, tend to show *lower basal cortisol levels* and a *blunted CAR* compared to typically developing peers [32, 34]. Angeli et al. [35] observed this particularly in children with the *combined* ADHD presentation, noting reduced cortisol both in the morning (30 minutes after waking) and in the evening, suggesting a *flatter overall profile* and potential *hypoarousal* [35]. Still, the data are not entirely consistent. Some studies on adults with ADHD show no significant difference in morning cortisol or CAR compared to controls, raising the possibility that this alteration may be *age-dependent* or *less pronounced over time* [36–39]. Other research adds nuance by *highlighting comorbidities*. For example, Imeraj et al. [33] found that children with ADHD but without oppositional defiant disorder (ODD) displayed morning hypoarousal and evening hyperarousal, while those with comorbid ODD showed the reverse pattern [33].

Different results might stem from variations *in study design* (e.g., single vs. repeated measures), sample *characteristics* (e.g., age and medication status), or *individual differences in HPA function*. That said, many researchers agree that reduced morning cortisol in ADHD tends to correlate with *delayed sleep phase* and *evening chronotype preferences* [40, 41]. Some studies suggest that the dampened cortisol rhythm may underpin the *motivational* and *cognitive energetic deficits observed* in ADHD, possibly as a consequence of dysregulation in the LCR and its interaction with the SCN [15, 33].

Higher cortisol levels have been observed among those with subclinical phenotypes, individuals who did not meet the criteria for a diagnosis of ADHD but showed *higher levels* of hyperactivity and/or inattention than other individuals in the population. It may represent a *previous stage* of HPA axis dysregulation, or alternatively, a consequence of *prolonged life stress* [42].

These findings on melatonin and cortisol support a larger model of ADHD being more than simply disrupted sleep [34]. Rather, this oscillatory abnormality could represent a worldwide circadian dysregulation, altering the neuroendocrine control and arousal states of the patient's everyday activities [33]. From this perspective, there are exciting opportunities to explore the biological underpinnings of this disorder that exist beyond the tight confines of the typical cognitive or behavioral spectrum [15].

This circadian dimension is *strongly supported* by converging *genetic, molecular, and neurobiological evidence* that core clock genes are involved in the pathophysiology of ADHD. The most robust findings is the association between the *3111 T/C single nucleotide polymorphism* in the 3′-untranslated region of the CLOCK gene and both ADHD, as well as the *delayed sleep phase syndrome* (DSPS). Multiple studies across diverse populations have shown that carriers of the T-allele exhibit a higher risk for ADHD, a stronger evening chronotype, and later sleep onset [27, 43, 44].

In addition to CLOCK, polymorphisms in other core circadian genes, *BMAL1* (ARNTL) and *PER2* have also been reported [40]. Studies have shown *lower rhythmic expression of these genes* in ADHD individuals, in which a *lower amplitude of PER2* was associated with higher severity of clinical symptoms, mainly for the inattentive clinical manifestation [27, 40].

To understand the functional impact of these genetic alterations, it is useful to examine the *molecular clock mechanism*. The CLOCK and BMAL1 proteins, both members of the basic helix-loop-helix PER-ARNT-SIM (bHLH-PAS) family form a heterodimer that acts as a transcriptional activator [15, 27, 45]. This complex binds to E-box elements present in the promoters of target genes, such as PER1, PER2, CRY1, and CRY2, activating their transcription [46]. The subsequent PER and CRY proteins dimerize and translocate back into the nucleus and inhibit the activity of the CLOCK:BMAL1 complex, effectively completing the *negative feedback loop* [45].

In parallel, a *second interlocked loop* involves the transcription of REV-ERBα/β and RORα/β, which regulate BMAL1 expression by binding to its promoter. *REV-ERBs act as repressors*, while *RORs function as activators*, providing additional rhythmic control [15, 27]. The evidence of animal studies supports these relationships. In spontaneously hypertensive rats (SHR) (an established model of ADHD) experimental perturbation of *PER1* and *CRY1* has been demonstrated to modulate behavior in a manner that is analogous to major ADHD symptoms, including hyperactivity and impaired impulse control [15, 27].

These genes are also of interest because they regulate *dopamine*, synthesis and release, thereby influencing *dopaminergic tone* in brain regions subserving attention, motivation, and impulse control [33]. Dysregulation of CLOCK, PER1, and PER2 can result in *altered dopaminergic rhythms*, a phenomenon that has also been implicated in the pathogenesis of manic symptoms in bipolar disorder, suggesting shared chronobiological mechanisms across distinct psychiatric conditions [47].

To add another layer, some scientists have suggested that people with ADHD might have changes in the function of the *LC*—a brainstem region that is critically important for attention and arousal *via* the norepinephrine system. In this model, the LC functions primarily in a *tonic mode* with reduced flexibility to switch to a *phasic, stimulus-driven mode* [33]. Such diminished flexibility could *compromise attending* to the environmental stimuli by updating focus and could thus be *related to the attentional problems* that are commonly present in ADHD [48].

Collectively, these data highlight that circadian dysregulation in ADHD affects several domains, from *sleep-wake timing* to *hormonal output* and *gene expression*. This unification of the chronobiological model not only advances our understanding of the pathophysiology of the disorder, but serves as the basis for other, more circumscribed, biologically based interventions.

2.2 Developmental trajectories and chronotype

The influence of circadian dysregulation in ADHD does not remain static throughout development. Its manifestations and clinical implications shift across age, shaped by physiological maturation and changing environmental demands.

In *early childhood*, the circadian system is still developing. Sleep-wake patterns at this stage are *highly responsive to external cues*, and disruptions can have pronounced effects. Some studies suggest that circadian misalignment may *worsen hyperactivity and impulsivity* in this age group. Imeraj et al. [33], for instance, describe "*paradoxical hyperactivity*," a pattern in which children exhibit increased daytime activity in response to underlying sleepiness, likely reflecting an *immature arousal regulation system* [33]

Bondopadhyay et al. [49], in a systematic review of children aged 5–13, found that those with ADHD were more likely to experience *sleep-onset difficulties, bedtime resistance*, and frequent *nocturnal awakenings* compared to their peers [49].

These sleep disturbances were closely tied to *externalizing behaviors*, such as *hyperactivity* and *oppositional tendencies*. In fact, poor sleep in this developmental stage has also been associated with *more severe ADHD symptoms* and a *higher risk for comorbid* mood *and anxiety disorders* later on [49, 50].

As children reach school age, the interaction between circadian timing and cognitive performance becomes more evident. Disruptions in sleep rhythms tend to manifest as *difficulties with attention, executive functioning*, and *academic learning* [51, 52]. Several studies document that children with ADHD and circadian rhythm disturbances demonstrate *poorer performance* on tasks requiring *sustained attention*, *working memory*, and *impulse control*, especially in the morning when their biological clocks may still be *misaligned with social demands* [46, 51, 53]. Actigraphy-based studies confirm that later chronotypes struggle more with *attentional control* in the morning and report higher levels *of daytime fatigue* [25].

Furthermore, Lunsford-Avery et al. [52] emphasize that in this age group, circadian misalignment is not just about sleep. It also *interferes* with *peer relationships* and *emotional regulation*, amplifying the overall burden of ADHD symptoms [52].

The *adolescent* years mark a critical shift. Due to natural physiological changes, teenagers tend to adopt *later sleep and wake times*. This phase delay often clashes with increasing academic demands, social pressures, and newfound autonomy over bedtime routines [54]. Adolescents with ADHD are especially vulnerable: they are more likely to develop *DSPS* and struggle with *sleep hygiene* [55].

This has *direct consequences* not just for sleep quality but also for mood stability, emotional reactivity, and attentional performance [46].

One important issue in adolescence is the interaction between *medication and circadian phase*. Stimulant medications have well-defined windows of peak effectiveness and side-effect profiles that are *highly sensitive to timing*. When circadian delays are present, optimal medication timing becomes harder to manage, potentially reducing benefits or amplifying adverse effects [15, 46, 56]. Again, Lunsford-Avery et al. [52] argue that aligning treatment with biological rhythms may offer real clinical advantages [52].

In *young adulthood*, external structures such as school timetables tend to disappear. Without these cues, many individuals with ADHD show even *greater variability* in their sleep-wake cycles. This irregularity can *destabilize circadian rhythms further*. Giannotta et al. [46] discuss how "*social jetlag*," a mismatch between biological and social time, can worsen ADHD symptoms and *reduce treatment efficacy* [46].

Bouteldja et al. [27] note that many young adults with ADHD exhibit a *delayed chronotype*, which is linked not only to poor sleep but also to increased *impulsivity*, emotional dysregulation, and risk-prone behavior [27]. Although some studies point to variability in sleep timing, the most consistent pattern remains a delayed phase. This shift is associated with *worse academic and occupational outcomes*, and reduced responsiveness to standard interventions [52, 57].

In sum, circadian vulnerabilities evolve across development. Recognizing how these patterns shift and how they interact with treatment, emotion, and cognition is essential for tailoring care. Future research should continue to map out these trajectories, ideally identifying those most likely to benefit from age-specific, rhythm-aligned interventions (**Figure 1**).

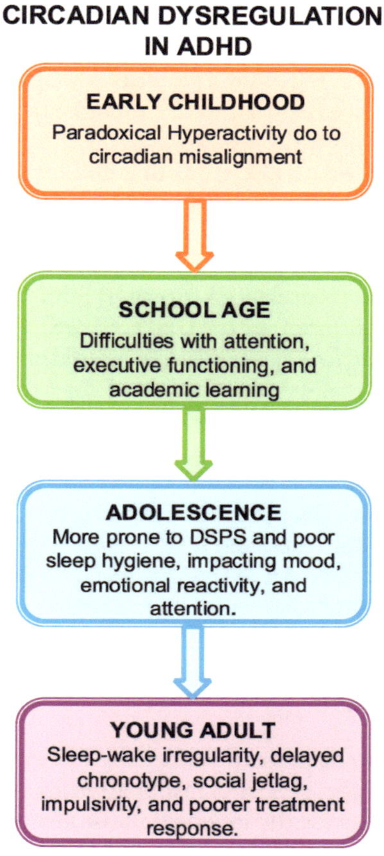

Figure 1.
Circadian dysregulation in ADHD across the lifespan.

2.3 Comorbidities in ADHD: The role of circadian and sleep dysfunctions

In individuals with ADHD, emotional regulation difficulties are common, and they often *overlap* with *mood disorders* such as depression, bipolar disorder, and cyclothymia [58]. These conditions share more than just clinical symptoms. Increasing evidence points to *disrupted circadian timing* as a common thread [40].

People with ADHD comorbid with mood instability often show delays in sleep onset, irregular melatonin production, or altered cortisol rhythms [26, 59]. These patterns *mirror* those seen in primary mood disorders, suggesting *shared physiological mechanisms* [33, 60]. As explained in Section 2.1, this often is due to a DLMO onset and an altered cortisol secretion pattern, indicating a larger circadian phase shift. These alterations at the physiological level may represent a *common substrate* for the attentional and *affective dysfunctions*. The more pronounced the circadian misalignment, the more severe the mood symptoms tend to be [27, 46].

Sleep fragmentation and poor sleep quality can *worsen both attention and affect regulation* [61]. In children and adolescents with ADHD, disrupted sleep may not only heighten irritability or impulsivity but also *increase vulnerability to anxiety and depression over time* [52]. This *bidirectional relationship* reinforces the need to look beyond core ADHD symptoms and consider circadian health as a potential intervention point [62].

What makes this even more relevant is that many of the same genes implicated in circadian regulation (CLOCK, BMAL1, PER, and CRY) have also been *linked to ADHD* and *mood disorders* [46, 63]. These genetic overlaps suggest that some individuals may be biologically predisposed to circadian instability, which in turn affects both mood and cognitive control [27, 46, 47].

About sleep disorders, research also finds that children with ADHD are far more likely to have *restless leg syndrome (RLS)*, which is an overwhelming urge to move the legs to relieve unpleasant, uncomfortable sensations, especially at rest [64]. This may in turn lead to both difficulties falling asleep and maintaining sleep. RLS leads to EMG disruptions in 1.5–2% of unselected (normal) children, while complaints are reported in almost 50% of children with ADHD [65, 66]. The overlap in pathogenesis, including *common neurobiological mechanisms* (e.g., midbrain dopamine dysfunction and frontal and prefrontal dysfunction), and shared *genetic* contributions might explain this association [67, 68]. Furthermore, the low levels of *serum ferritin*, which is frequently found in children with ADHD, have been found to be associated with RLS, which may be related to the fact that iron is a cofactor in dopamine synthesis [64, 69]. Other problems with sleep, including *obstructive sleep apnea* and *delayed sleep phase syndrome*, are also widely reported in kids with ADHD [64].

Stabilizing circadian rhythms could therefore serve a dual purpose: improving ADHD-related symptoms while also reducing emotional dysregulation, comorbid mood disturbances, and sleep disorders.

2.4 Circadian rhythms and pharmacotherapy

The intricate relationship between the circadian system and the pharmacological management of ADHD has garnered increasing attention in the scientific literature. The circadian system is also critically involved in the absorption, metabolism, and efficacy of medications, including those used for ADHD [70, 71].

The *timing of drug administration* in relation to an individual's circadian phase can affect drug *absorption, metabolism, and elimination*, ultimately impacting efficacy and the risk of *adverse effects* [46, 72, 73]. In individuals with ADHD, who typically exhibit a delayed circadian phase and evening chronotype, the administration of stimulant medications such as *methylphenidate* (MPH) or *amphetamines later in the day* may *exacerbate sleep-onset difficulties, prolong sleep latency*, and *reduce sleep duration* [56, 73–75].

As mentioned in *Section 2.1*, this chronotype is related to a DLMO and sometimes to abnormal melatonin metabolism, conditions which could shorten the temporal period of efficacy both of hormonal and pharmacological treatments. These circadian misalignments may also have the potential to diminish the efficacy of ADHD medications and increase the risk for sleep related side effects.

Disrupted circadian rhythms can also *alter hepatic enzyme activity* involved in drug metabolism, leading to interindividual variability in drug exposure and response [46]. For instance, evening dosing of stimulants may result in *higher plasma concentrations* during the biological night, when metabolic clearance is reduced, increasing the risk of *insomnia* and other *stimulant-induced side effects* [72, 76, 77].

Alterations in sleep patterns, including *sleep deprivation* and *delayed or disrupted melatonin rhythms*, are highly prevalent in individuals with ADHD and are frequently observed *even before the initiation of pharmacological treatment* [24, 25, 62, 74, 78]. *Sleep loss* itself can impair executive functioning, mood regulation, and attentional control, thereby compounding the core symptoms of ADHD and potentially *attenuating the benefits of stimulant medications* [76, 78–81]. Moreover, sleep deprivation has been shown to *disrupt the function of the dopaminergic system* (one of the principal targets of stimulant therapy) suggesting a neurobiological mechanism by which poor sleep *may reduce medication efficacy* [24, 76, 81].

Melatonin release delay could interact with the *pharmacodynamics* of both stimulant and non-stimulant treatments. For example, *exogenous melatonin administration in the evening* has been shown to *advance sleep onset* and *improve sleep quality* in children with ADHD experiencing stimulant-induced insomnia, demonstrating the therapeutic potential of aligning pharmacotherapy with circadian biology [60, 79].

Meta-analyses and clinical trials have yielded mixed results regarding the impact of stimulants on sleep. Some studies report that *stimulants increase sleep latency* and *reduce total sleep time*, particularly during the initial weeks of treatment or following dose escalation [56, 73, 77, 78, 82]. For example, in a meta-analysis of nine studies, stimulant use in children and adolescents was associated with moderately reduced total sleep duration, delayed sleep onset, and decreased sleep efficiency [83].

Conversely, other studies have found *neutral* or even *positive effects* of stimulants on sleep, especially when ADHD symptoms such as hyperactivity and bedtime resistance are *ameliorated*, facilitating a *more consistent sleep routine* [25, 49, 52]. Notably, actigraphy-based studies in adults have reported that methylphenidate may *improve sleep efficiency* and *reduce nocturnal motor activity*, particularly after a period of treatment stabilization [75].

The heterogeneity in findings is likely attributable to several factors, including differences in study design, medication dose and formulation, time of administration, and the presence of baseline sleep or circadian disturbances [6, 49]. Importantly, individuals with preexisting sleep problems appear to be at greater risk for stimulant-induced sleep disturbances [81].

Non-stimulant treatments for ADHD, such as atomoxetine (a selective norepinephrine reuptake inhibitor), guanfacine, and clonidine (alpha-2 adrenergic agonists), offer alternative therapeutic options, particularly for patients who do not tolerate stimulants or have comorbidities [84, 85]. *Atomoxetine* has been associated with *less pronounced negative effects on sleep* compared to stimulants and, in some cases, may improve sleep onset latency and reduce insomnia symptoms [72, 86, 87]. Nevertheless, even non-stimulant medications can influence circadian rhythms. Animal studies indicate that *atomoxetine* can *phase-shift* the circadian clock and alter clock gene expression [88, 89]. Clinical observations suggest that the *sedative properties of alpha-2 agonists* may be beneficial in ADHD patients with *prominent sleep-onset difficulties*, though daytime somnolence and other adverse effects require careful monitoring [86, 90].

ADHD frequently *co-occurs with other psychiatric disorders*, including *mood* and *anxiety disorders*, as well as *sleep* and *circadian rhythm disturbances* [24, 91]. Metabolic comorbidities, such as *obesity* and *insulin resistance*, are also more prevalent among individuals with ADHD and are themselves *influenced by circadian misalignment* [26, 32, 33]. These comorbidities not only complicate treatment selection but also further *increase the risk of sleep problems and medication side effects* [80, 92].

Given this complexity, a *personalized* approach to ADHD management is paramount. *Chronotherapeutic strategies*—such as aligning medication timing with individual circadian profiles, utilizing melatonin or light therapy to advance circadian phase, and implementing behavioral sleep interventions—may *enhance treatment efficacy* and *minimize adverse effects* [15, 46, 62].

The interplay between the circadian system and ADHD pharmacotherapy is complex and clinically significant. Circadian disruption can alter the metabolism and efficacy of stimulant and non-stimulant medications, with downstream effects on sleep, mood, and metabolic health. Sleep deprivation and melatonin dysregulation further limit the benefits of treatment and increase the risk of adverse events. The frequent coexistence of ADHD with sleep, mood, and metabolic disorders further underscores the necessity of individualized, chronobiologically informed care. Future research and clinical practice should prioritize the integration of circadian assessment and intervention into ADHD management to optimize outcomes and quality of life for affected individuals.

2.5 Intervention in circadian rhythm disruptions

Interest in interventions targeting circadian disruptions in ADHD has grown significantly in recent years. Among the most promising strategies are *chronotherapeutic approaches* such as light therapy, melatonin supplementation, and structured behavioral treatments [27, 46, 60, 70].

Light therapy, for example, has been shown to advance the circadian phase in adults with ADHD, with more pronounced *phase shifts* correlating with stronger symptom improvements [93]. Similarly, *melatonin treatment* appears particularly effective in children suffering from sleep-onset insomnia. It not only advances DLMO but also shortens sleep latency and improves sleep quality, especially in those with delayed chronotypes [94, 95].

Meta-analyses and systematic reviews confirm these results, showing that melatonin can reliably *improve both sleep onset and duration in pediatric ADHD* populations and does so with relatively few side effects [96, 97].

Behavioral interventions also hold value. Techniques like *sleep hygiene education* and *behavioral sleep therapy* have been linked not only to improved sleep patterns but also to *moderate reductions in ADHD symptom severity* [57, 98]. Still, the *current evidence base remains limited*: many studies are small, varied in method, and not always reproducible. There is a clear need for more robust randomized trials, ideally incorporating "chrono-diagnostic" methods to tailor treatment to the individual's circadian profile [15].

Timing also matters. Recent research underscores that both stimulant and non-stimulant ADHD medications can *interact with circadian dynamics*, sometimes helping, sometimes disrupting them [73, 82]. *Aligning* drug administration with the individual's biological clock could significantly *improve both efficacy and tolerability* [27, 46, 60, 70].

While melatonin offers the strongest evidence base in children, light therapy demonstrates substantial promise in adults, though its clinical use remains limited by practical barriers. Behavioral strategies, meanwhile, stand out for their sustainability and minimal adverse effects, despite a comparatively weaker body of evidence [94].

In sum, chronotherapy represents a promising, biologically grounded path for *managing ADHD-related sleep and arousal issues*. But to move from promise to practice, we need larger, better-designed studies and a deeper understanding of individual circadian phenotypes [94].

3. Conclusion

In sum, substantial data supports the idea of circadian dysfunction having an important role in the *etiology*, *course*, and *presentation* of ADHD. This chronobiological liability, typically expressed as *delayed sleep phase*, *abnormal melatonin secretion*, and *disturbed rest-activity rhythms*, not only contributes to the *characteristic symptoms* of inattention and impulsivity but also to the common *emotional lability* and *comorbid* mood disorders found in those with ADHD.

These results have important clinical implications. Traditional treatments of ADHD, which primarily focus on behavioral symptoms and pharmacotherapy with stimulants, commonly overlook the underlying circadian foundation of the disorder that can facilitate the onset of symptoms or perturb the response to therapies. Disregarding the patient-specific circadian phase when applying drug schedules may lead to *reduced efficacy* of treatment and may result in *side effects* such as insomnia, agitation, and rebound phenomena. *In contrast*, sleep hygiene, melatonin, or light therapy to adjust the circadian phase, or optimization of medicine timing with respect to the *circadian phase*, offer the opportunity to provide these patients with many more hours of *symptom control* and *functional well-being*.

Personalized chronotherapeutics represents a transformation in the treatment of ADHD. Instead of a "one-size-fits-all" approach, circadian profiling can be incorporated into clinical interviews, actigraphy, sleep logs, or biological factors when considering diagnoses and treatment approaches. This level of *personalization* not only could *increase treatment adherence* and *tolerability* but could also *mitigate the need for high-dose medication* by targeting upstream bodily dysregulations. This approach is especially suitable for patients with prominent sleep problems, treatment resistance, or complicated comorbidities such as anxiety or bipolar spectrum symptoms.

For future studies, circadian/sleep patterns could be included as a part of standard ADHD evaluation in clinical protocols. The research that follows should further refine these trials, emphasizing studies that investigate as well as test across developmental epochs multimodal, circadian-based treatment regimens. In the end, making biological rhythms a *focus of care* might enable clinicians to provide more effective, longer-lasting, and personalized results for those with ADHD.

Conflict of interest

The authors declare no conflict of interest.

Nomenclature

ADHD	attention-deficit/hyperactivity disorder
CRD	circadian rhythm dysregulation
SCN	suprachiasmatic nucleus
HPA axis	hypothalamic-pituitary-adrenal axis
LC	locus coeruleus
DSPS	delayed sleep phase syndrome
DSPD	delayed sleep phase disorder
DLMO	dim light melatonin onset
CAR	cortisol awakening response
MEQ	morningness–eveningness questionnaire
MCTQ	munich chronotype questionnaire
TST	total sleep time
SOL	sleep onset latency
WASO	wake after sleep onset

CLOCK	gene encoding a transcription factor that initiates circadian rhythms
BMAL1	gene encoding the partner of CLOCK in the core circadian transcriptional loop
PER1/PER2	genes encoding PER proteins, which inhibit CLOCK:BMAL1 activity
CRY1/CRY2	genes encoding CRY proteins, part of the negative feedback loop
REV-ERBα/β	nuclear receptor genes repressing BMAL1 transcription
RORα/β	nuclear receptor genes activating BMAL1 transcription
bHLH-PAS	protein family (basic helix-loop-helix-PER-ARNT-SIM) involved in circadian gene regulation
EEG	electroencephalography
RLS	restless legs syndrome
SHR	spontaneously hypertensive rat (ADHD animal model)
MPH	methylphenidate
SNP	single nucleotide polymorphism

Author details

Alessandra Carta*, Vanna Cavassa and Stefano Sotgiu
Division of Child Neuropsychiatry, University Hospital of Sassari (AOU SASSARI)-Department of Medicine, Surgery and Pharmacy, University of Sassari, Sassari, Italy

*Address all correspondence to: alessandra.carta@aouss.it

References

[1] Goldschmied JR, Palermo E, Yocum A, McInnis M, Gehrman P. The relationship between sleep and circadian patterns with risk for suicide in bipolar disorder varies by subtype. Journal of Psychiatric Research. 2025;**181**:23-28

[2] Deprato A, Haldar P, Navarro JF, Harding BN, Lacy P, Maidstone R, et al. Associations between light at night and mental health: A systematic review and meta-analysis. Science of the Total Environment. 2025;**974**:179188

[3] Mendoza Alvarez M, Balthasar Y, Verbraecken J, Claes L, van Someren E, van Marle HJF, et al. Systematic review: REM sleep, dysphoric dreams and nightmares as transdiagnostic features of psychiatric disorders with emotion dysregulation - clinical implications. Sleep Medicine. 2025;**127**:1-15

[4] Bromundt V. Circadian rhythm sleep disorders in psychiatric diseases. Therapeutische Umschau. Revue Therapeutique. 2014;**71**(11):663-670

[5] van der Ham M, Bijlenga D, Böhmer M, Beekman ATF, Kooij S. Sleep problems in adults with ADHD: Prevalences and their relationship with psychiatric comorbidity. Journal of Attention Disorders. 2024;**28**(13):1642-1652

[6] Faraone SV, Bellgrove MA, Brikell I, Cortese S, Hartman CA, Hollis C, et al. Attention-deficit/hyperactivity disorder. Nature Reviews Disease Primers. 2024;**10**(1):1-21

[7] Arildskov TW, Thomsen PH, Sonuga-Barke EJS, Lambek R, Østergaard SD, Virring A. Is attention-deficit/hyperactivity disorder (ADHD) a dimension or a category? What does the relationship between ADHD traits and psychosocial quality of life tell us? Journal of Attention Disorders. 2024;**28**(7):1035-1044

[8] Borbély AA. A two process model of sleep regulation. Human Neurobiology. 1982;**1**(3):195-204

[9] Siegel JM. Clues to the functions of mammalian sleep. Nature. 2005;**437**(7063):1264-1271

[10] Aschoff J, Wever R. Human circadian rhythms: A multioscillatory system. Federation Proceedings. 1976;**35**(12):236-232

[11] Herljevic M, Middleton B, Thapan K, Skene DJ. Light-induced melatonin suppression: Age-related reduction in response to short wavelength light. Experimental Gerontology. 2005;**40**(3):237-242

[12] Eisenstein M. Chronobiology: Stepping out of time. Nature. 2013;**497**(7450):S10-S12

[13] Ardura J, Gutierrez R, Andres J, Agapito T. Emergence and evolution of the circadian rhythm of melatonin in children. Hormone Research. 2003;**59**(2):66-72

[14] Breen S, Rees S, Walker D. The development of diurnal rhythmicity in fetal suprachiasmatic neurons as demonstrated by fos immunohistochemistry. Neuroscience. 1996;**74**(3):917-926

[15] Coogan AN, Baird AL, Popa-Wagner A, Thome J. Circadian rhythms and attention deficit hyperactivity disorder: The what, the when and the why. Progress in

Neuro-Psychopharmacology & Biological Psychiatry. 2016;**67**:74-81

[16] Baser KHC, Haskologlu IC, Erdag E. Molecular links between circadian rhythm disruption, melatonin, and neurodegenerative diseases: An updated review. Molecules Basel Switzerland. 2025;**30**(9):1888

[17] Chen Y, Liu P, Sabo A, Guan D. Human genetic variation determines 24-hour rhythmic gene expression and disease risk. Nature Communications. 2025;**16**(1):4270

[18] Niu L, Gao Q, Xie M, Yip T, Gunnar MR, Wang W, et al. Association of childhood adversity with HPA axis activity in children and adolescents: A systematic review and meta-analysis. Neuroscience and Biobehavioral Reviews. 2025;**172**:106124

[19] Becker SP, Luebbe AM, Kofler MJ, Burns GL, Jarrett MA. ADHD, chronotype, and circadian preference in a multi-site sample of college students. Journal of Sleep Research. 2024;**33**(1):e13994

[20] Martinez-Cayuelas E, Moreno-Vinues B, Pozo RLD, Rodrigo-Moreno M, Soto-Insuga V, Pérez-Villena A. Sleep, chronotype, and behavior in adolescents with attention-deficit/hyperactivity disorder. Archives of Pediatrie Organe Officiel Societe Francaise Pediatrics. 2022;**29**(4):277-280

[21] Coogan AN, McGowan NM. A systematic review of circadian function, chronotype and chronotherapy in attention deficit hyperactivity disorder. Attention deficit hyperactivity disorder. 2017;**9**(3):129-147

[22] Taillard J, Sagaspe P, Philip P, Bioulac S. Sleep timing, chronotype and social jetlag: Impact on cognitive abilities and psychiatric disorders. Biochemical Pharmacology. 2021;**191**:114438

[23] Coleman MY, Cain SW. Eveningness is associated with greater subjective cognitive impairment in individuals with self-reported symptoms of unipolar depression. Journal of Affective Disorders. 2019;**256**:404-415

[24] Yoon SYR, Jain U, Shapiro C. Sleep in attention-deficit/hyperactivity disorder in children and adults: Past, present, and future. Sleep Medicine Reviews. 2012;**16**(4):371-388

[25] Ziegler M, Kaiser A, Igel C, Geissler J, Mechler K, Holz NE, et al. Actigraphy-derived sleep profiles of children with and without attention-deficit/hyperactivity disorder (ADHD) over two weeks—Comparison, precursor symptoms, and the chronotype. Brain Sciences. 2021;**11**(12):1564

[26] Van Veen MM, Kooij JJS, Boonstra AM, Gordijn MCM, Van Someren EJW. Delayed circadian rhythm in adults with attention-deficit/hyperactivity disorder and chronic sleep-onset insomnia. Biological Psychiatry. 2010;**67**(11):1091-1096

[27] Bouteldja AA, Penichet D, Srivastava LK, Cermakian N. The circadian system: A neglected player in neurodevelopmental disorders. The European Journal of Neuroscience. 2024;**60**(2):3858-3890

[28] Büber A, Çakaloz B, Işıldar Y, Ünlü G, Bostancı HE, Aybek H, et al. Increased urinary 6-hydroxymelatoninsulfate levels in attention deficit hyperactivity disorder diagnosed children and adolescent. Neuroscience Letters. 2016;**617**:195-200

[29] Predescu E, Vaidean T, Rapciuc AM, Sipos R. Metabolomic markers in attention-deficit/hyperactivity disorder

(ADHD) among children and adolescents—A systematic review. International Journal of Molecular Sciences. 2024;**25**(8):4385

[30] Van Cauter E, Désir D, Decoster C, Féry F, Balasse EO. Nocturnal decrease in glucose tolerance during constant glucose infusion. The Journal of Clinical Endocrinology and Metabolism. 1989;**69**(3):604-611

[31] Van Cauter E, Polonsky KS, Scheen AJ. Roles of circadian rhythmicity and sleep in human glucose regulation. Endocrine Reviews. 1997;**18**(5):716-738

[32] Van Andel E, Vogel SWN, Bijlenga D, Kalsbeek A, Beekman ATF, Kooij JJS. Effects of chronotherapeutic interventions in adults with ADHD and delayed sleep phase syndrome (DSPS) on regulation of appetite and glucose metabolism. Journal of Attention Disorders. 2024;**28**(13):1653-1667

[33] Imeraj L, Sonuga-Barke E, Antrop I, Roeyers H, Wiersema R, Bal S, et al. Altered circadian profiles in attention-deficit/hyperactivity disorder: An integrative review and theoretical framework for future studies. Neuroscience and Biobehavioral Reviews. 2012;**36**(8):1897-1919

[34] Chang JPC, Su KP, Mondelli V, Pariante CM. Cortisol and inflammatory biomarker levels in youths with attention deficit hyperactivity disorder (ADHD): Evidence from a systematic review with meta-analysis. Translational Psychiatry. 2021;**11**:430

[35] Angeli E, Korpa T, Johnson EO, Apostolakou F, Papassotiriou I, Chrousos GP, et al. Salivary cortisol and alpha-amylase diurnal profiles and stress reactivity in children with attention deficit hyperactivity disorder. Psychoneuroendocrinology. 2018;**90**:174-181

[36] Bonvicini C, Faraone SV, Scassellati C. Common and specific genes and peripheral biomarkers in children and adults with attention-deficit/hyperactivity disorder. World Journal of Biological Psychiatry Officie Journal of World Federation of Societies of Biological Psychiatry. 2018;**19**(2):80-100

[37] Hirvikoski T, Lindholm T, Nordenström A, Nordström AL, Lajic S. High self-perceived stress and many stressors, but normal diurnal cortisol rhythm, in adults with ADHD (attention-deficit/hyperactivity disorder). Hormones and Behavior. 2009;**55**(3):418-424

[38] Ramos-Quiroga JA, Corominas-Roso M, Palomar G, Ferrer R, Valero S, Corrales M, et al. Cortisol awakening response in adults with attention deficit hyperactivity disorder: Subtype differences and association with the emotional lability. European Neuropsychopharmacology Journal of the European College of Neuropsychopharmacology. 2016;**26**(7):1140-1149

[39] Carta A, Vainieri I, Rommel AS, Zuddas A, Kuntsi J, Sotgiu S, et al. Temperament dimensions and awakening cortisol levels in attention-deficit/hyperactivity disorder. Frontiers in Psychiatry. 2022;**13**:803001

[40] Baird AL, Coogan AN, Siddiqui A, Donev RM, Thome J. Adult attention-deficit hyperactivity disorder is associated with alterations in circadian rhythms at the behavioural, endocrine and molecular levels. Molecular Psychiatry. 2012;**17**(10):988-995

[41] Randler C, Schaal S. Morningness-eveningness, habitual sleep-wake variables and cortisol level. Biological Psychology. 2010;**85**(1):14-18

[42] Berens A, LeMoult J, Kircanski K, Gotlib IH. ADHD symptoms and diurnal cortisol in adolescents: The importance of comorbidities. Psychoneuroendocrinology. 2023;**148**:105990

[43] Kissling C, Retz W, Wiemann S, Coogan AN, Clement RM, Hünnerkopf R, et al. A polymorphism at the 3′-untranslated region of the CLOCK gene is associated with adult attention-deficit hyperactivity disorder. American Journal of Medical Genetics Part B: Neuropsychiatric Genetics: The Official Publication of the International Society of Psychiatric Genetics. 2008;**147**(3):333-338

[44] Xu X, Breen G, Chen CK, Huang YS, Wu YY, Asherson P. Association study between a polymorphism at the 3′-untranslated region of CLOCK gene and attention deficit hyperactivity disorder. Behavioral and Brain Functions. 2010;**6**:48

[45] Korshunov KS, Blakemore LJ, Trombley PQ. Dopamine: A modulator of circadian rhythms in the central nervous system. Frontiers in Cellular Neuroscience. 2017;**11**:91. Disponibile su: https://www.frontiersin.org/journals/cellular-neuroscience/articles/10.3389/fncel.2017.00091/full

[46] Giannotta G, Ruggiero M, Trabacca A. Chronobiology in paediatric neurological and neuropsychiatric disorders: Harmonizing care with biological clocks. Journal of Clinical Medicine. 2024;**13**(24):7737

[47] Quaranta G, Barbuti M, Pallucchini A, Colombini P, Moriconi M, Gemmellaro T, et al. Relationships among delayed sleep phase disorder, emotional dysregulation, and affective temperaments in adults with attention deficit hyperactivity disorder and cyclothymia. The Journal of Nervous and Mental Disease. 2020;**208**(11):857

[48] Speyer LG, Brown RH, Ribeaud D, Eisner M, Murray AL. The role of moment-to-moment dynamics of perceived stress and negative affect in co-occurring ADHD and internalising symptoms. Journal of Autism and Developmental Disorders. 2023;**53**(3):1213-1223

[49] Bondopadhyay U, Diaz-Orueta U, Coogan AN. A systematic review of sleep and circadian rhythms in children with attention deficit hyperactivity disorder. Journal of Attention Disorders. 2022;**26**(2):149-224

[50] Morales-Muñoz I, Upthegrove R, Lawrence K, Thayakaran R, Kooij S, Gregory AM, et al. The role of inflammation in the prospective associations between early childhood sleep problems and ADHD at 10 years: Findings from a UK birth cohort study. Journal of Child Psychology and Psychiatry. 2023;**64**(6):930-940

[51] Qu X, Kalb LG, Holingue C, Rojo-Wissar DM, Pritchard A, Spira AP, et al. Association of Time in bed, social jetlag and sleep disturbances with cognitive performance in children with ADHD. Journal of Attention Disorders. 2024;**28**(1):99-108

[52] Lunsford-Avery JR, Krystal AD, Kollins SH. Sleep disturbances in adolescents with ADHD: A systematic review and framework for future research. Clinical Psychology Review. 2016;**50**:159-174

[53] Becker SP. ADHD and sleep: Recent advances and future directions. Current Opinion in Psychology. 2020;**34**:50-56

[54] Carskadon MA. Sleep in adolescents: The perfect storm. Pediatric Clinics of North America. 2011;**58**(3):637-647

[55] Gruber R, Salamon L, Tauman R, Al-Yagon M. Sleep disturbances in

adolescents with attention-deficit/hyperactivity disorder. Nature and Science of Sleep. 2023;**15**:275-286

[56] Wiggs KK, Breaux R, Langberg JM, Peugh JL, Becker SP. Examining daily stimulant medication use and sleep in adolescents with ADHD. European Child & Adolescent Psychiatry. 2024;**33**(3):821-832

[57] Becker SP, Kapadia DK, Fershtman CEM, Sciberras E. Evening circadian preference is associated with sleep problems and daytime sleepiness in adolescents with ADHD. Journal of Sleep Research. 2020;**29**(1):e12936

[58] French B, Nalbant G, Wright H, Sayal K, Daley D, Groom MJ, et al. The impacts associated with having ADHD: An umbrella review. Frontiers in Psychiatry. 2024;**15**:1343314

[59] Spera V, Maiello M, Pallucchini A, Novi M, Elefante C, De Dominicis F, et al. Adult attention-deficit hyperactivity disorder and clinical correlates of delayed sleep phase disorder. Psychiatry Research. 2020;**291**:113162

[60] Moon E, Kim K, Partonen T, Linnaranta O. Role of melatonin in the management of sleep and circadian disorders in the context of psychiatric illness. Current Psychiatry Reports. 2022;**24**(11):623-634

[61] van der Helm E, Gujar N, Walker MP. Sleep deprivation impairs the accurate recognition of human emotions. Sleep. 2010;**33**(3):335-342

[62] Lunsford-Avery JR, Davis JL, Willoughby MT. Circadian rhythm dysfunction and clinical heterogeneity in pediatric ADHD: A critical need for innovation in assessment and treatment. JCPP Advances. 2024;**5**(1):e12281

[63] Waddington Lamont E, Legault-Coutu D, Cermakian N, Boivin DB. The role of circadian clock genes in mental disorders. Dialogues in Clinical Neuroscience. 2007;**9**(3):333-342

[64] Belli A, Breda M, Di Maggio C, Esposito D, Marcucci L, Bruni O. Children with neurodevelopmental disorders: How do they sleep? Current Opinion in Psychiatry. 2022;**35**(5):345

[65] Cortese S, Konofal E, Lecendreux M, Arnulf I, Mouren MC, Darra F, et al. Restless legs syndrome and attention-deficit/hyperactivity disorder: A review of the literature. Sleep. 2005;**28**(8):1007-1013

[66] DelRosso LM, Picchietti DL, Spruyt K, Bruni O, Garcia-Borreguero D, Kotagal S, et al. Restless sleep in children: A systematic review. Sleep Medicine Reviews. 2021;**56**:101406

[67] Didriksen M, Thørner LW, Erikstrup C, Pedersen OB, Paarup HM, Petersen M, et al. Self-reported restless legs syndrome and involuntary leg movements during sleep are associated with symptoms of attention deficit hyperactivity disorder. Sleep Medicine. 2019;**57**:115-121

[68] Schimmelmann BG, Friedel S, Nguyen TT, Sauer S, Ganz Vogel CI, Konrad K, et al. Exploring the genetic link between RLS and ADHD. Journal of Psychiatric Research. 2009;**43**(10):941-945

[69] Konofal E, Cortese S, Marchand M, Mouren MC, Arnulf I, Lecendreux M. Impact of restless legs syndrome and iron deficiency on attention-deficit/hyperactivity disorder in children. Sleep Medicine. 2007;**8**(7-8):711-715

[70] Coogan AN, Schenk M, Palm D, Uzoni A, Grube J, Tsang AH, et al. Impact of adult attention deficit hyperactivity disorder and medication status on sleep/wake behavior and molecular circadian

rhythms. Neuropsychopharmacology, the Official Publication of the American College of Neuropsychopharmacology. 2019;**44**(7):1198-1206

[71] Boonstra AM, Kooij JJS, Oosterlaan J, Sergeant JA, Buitelaar JK, Van Someren EJW. Hyperactive night and day? Actigraphy studies in adult ADHD: A baseline comparison and the effect of methylphenidate. Sleep. 2007;**30**(4):433-442

[72] Faraone SV, Banaschewski T, Coghill D, Zheng Y, Biederman J, Bellgrove MA, et al. The world federation of ADHD international consensus statement: 208 evidence-based conclusions about the disorder. Neuroscience and Biobehavioral Reviews. 2021;**128**:789-818

[73] Cataldo M, Donnelly G, Cutler AJ, Childress A, Mikl J, Bhaskar S, et al. Analysis of daily sleep diary measures from multilayer extended-release methylphenidate (PRC-063) studies in children and adults with ADHD. Journal of Attention Disorders. 2022;**26**(14):1870-1881

[74] Checa-Ros A, Muñoz-Hoyos A, Molina-Carballo A, Viejo-Boyano I, Chacín M, Bermúdez V, et al. Low doses of melatonin to improve sleep in children with ADHD: An open-label trial. Children. 2023;**10**(7):1121

[75] Fredriksen M, Golparian N, Beiske K, Stavem K. Impact of methylphenidate on sleep problems in adults with ADHD: A pilot polysomnography study. Nordic Journal of Psychiatry. 2021;**75**(3):234-238

[76] Corkum P, Begum EA, Rusak B, Rajda M, Shea S, MacPherson M et al. The Effects of Extended-Release Stimulant Medication on sleep in children with ADHD. Journal of the Canadian Academy of Child and Adolescent Psychiatry. Mar 2020;**29**(1):33-41

[77] Storebø OJ, Storm MRO, Pereira Ribeiro J, Skoog M, Groth C, Callesen HE, et al. Methylphenidate for children and adolescents with attention deficit hyperactivity disorder (ADHD). Cochrane Database of Systematic Reviews. 2023;**2023**(3):CD009885

[78] Weiss MD, Surman C, Khullar A, He E, Cataldo M, Donnelly G. Effect of a multi-layer, extended-release methylphenidate formulation (PRC-063) on sleep in adults with ADHD: A randomized, double-blind, forced-dose, placebo-controlled trial followed by a 6-month open-label extension. CNS Drugs. 2021;**35**(6):667-679

[79] Masi G, Fantozzi P, Villafranca A, Tacchi A, Ricci F, Ruglioni L, et al. Effects of melatonin in children with attention-deficit/hyperactivity disorder with sleep disorders after methylphenidate treatment. Neuropsychiatric Disease and Treatment. 2019;**15**:663-667

[80] Wajszilber D, Santiseban JA, Gruber R. Sleep disorders in patients with ADHD: Impact and management challenges. Nature and Science of Sleep. 2018;**10**:453-480

[81] D'Aiello B, Gessi L, Menghini D, Vicari S, De Rossi P. Sleep disturbances in children with ADHD on methylphenidate monotherapy: The role of dysregulation profile. Sleep Medicine. 2025;**128**:153-158

[82] Kidwell KM, Van Dyk TR, Lundahl A, Nelson TD. Stimulant medications and sleep for youth with ADHD: A meta-analysis. Pediatrics. 2015;**136**(6):1144-1153

[83] Denyer H, Carr E, Deng Q, Asherson P, Bilbow A, Folarin A, et al.

A 10-week remote monitoring study of sleep features and their variability in individuals with and without ADHD. BMC Psychiatry. 2025;**25**:294

[84] Ostinelli EG, Schulze M, Zangani C, Farhat LC, Tomlinson A, Del Giovane C, et al. Comparative efficacy and acceptability of pharmacological, psychological, and neurostimulatory interventions for ADHD in adults: A systematic review and component network meta-analysis. Lancet Psychiatry. 2025;**12**(1):32-43

[85] Farhat LC, Behling E, Landeros-Weisenberger A, Ferreira M, de Barros P, Polanczyk GV, et al. Pharmacological interventions for attention-deficit/hyperactivity disorder in children and adolescents with Tourette disorder: A systematic review and network meta-analysis. Journal of Child and Adolescent Psychopharmacology. 2024;**34**(9):373-382

[86] Rocha NS, Correa RDESA, Dias ACDM, Bueno CDF. Association between sleep pattern and pharmacological treatment in children with attention deficit disorder with hyperactivity: A systematic review. Revista Paulista de Pediatria. 2023;**41**:e2022065

[87] Burguete E, Peydro L, Ventura I. Bioethical evaluation of methylphenidate and atomoxetine for pediatric ADHD and cognitive enhancement. Philosophy, Ethics, and Humanities in Medicine. 2025;**20**(1):5

[88] O'Keeffe SM, Thome J, Coogan AN. The noradrenaline reuptake inhibitor atomoxetine phase-shifts the circadian clock in mice. Neuroscience. 2012;**201**:219-230

[89] Baird AL, Coogan AN, Kaufling J, Barrot M, Thome J. Daily methylphenidate and atomoxetine treatment impacts on clock gene protein expression in the mouse brain. Brain Research. 2013;**1513**:61-71

[90] Connor DF, Findling RL, Kollins SH, Sallee F, López FA, Lyne A, et al. Effects of guanfacine extended release on oppositional symptoms in children aged 6-12 years with attention-deficit hyperactivity disorder and oppositional symptoms: A randomized, double-blind, placebo-controlled trial. CNS Drugs. 2010;**24**(9):755-768

[91] Wynchank D, ten Have M, Bijlenga D, Penninx BW, Beekman AT, Lamers F, et al. The association between insomnia and sleep duration in adults with attention-deficit hyperactivity disorder: Results from a general population study. Journal of Clinical Sleep Medicine JCSM: Official American Academy of Sleep Medicine Journal. 2018;**14**(3):349-357

[92] Uygur H. Unraveling the insomnia puzzle: Sleep reactivity, attention deficit hyperactivity symptoms, and insomnia severity in ADHD patients. Frontiers in Psychiatry. 2025;**15**:1528979

[93] Rybak YE, McNeely HE, Mackenzie BE, Jain UR, Levitan RD. An open trial of light therapy in adult attention-deficit/hyperactivity disorder. The Journal of Clinical Psychiatry. 2006;**67**(10):1527-1535

[94] Cortese S, Fusetto Veronesi G, Gabellone A, Margari A, Marzulli L, Matera E, et al. The management of sleep disturbances in children with attention-deficit/hyperactivity disorder (ADHD): An update of the literature. Expert Review of Neurotherapeutics. 2024;**24**(6):585-596

[95] van der Heijden KB, Smits MG, Gunning WB. Sleep-related disorders in ADHD: A review. Clinical Pediatrics (Phila). 2005;**44**(3):201-210

[96] Salanitro M, Wrigley T, Ghabra H, de Haan E, Hill CM, Solmi M, et al. Efficacy on sleep parameters and tolerability of melatonin in individuals with sleep or mental disorders: A systematic review and meta-analysis. Neuroscience and Biobehavioral Reviews. 2022;**139**:104723

[97] Mombelli S, Bacaro V, Curati S, Berra F, Sforza M, Castronovo V, et al. Non-pharmacological and melatonin interventions for pediatric sleep initiation and maintenance problems: A systematic review and network meta-analysis. Sleep Medicine Reviews. 2023;**70**:101806

[98] Hiscock H, Sciberras E, Mensah F, Gerner B, Efron D, Khano S, et al. Impact of a behavioural sleep intervention on symptoms and sleep in children with attention deficit hyperactivity disorder, and parental mental health: Randomised controlled trial. BMJ. 2015;**350**:h68

Chapter 4

Sleep and ADHD

Martina Gnazzo, Valentina Baldini, Giulia Santangelo, Giuditta Bargiacchi and Marco Carotenuto

Abstract

Attention-Deficit/Hyperactivity Disorder (ADHD) is a neurodevelopmental disorder that affects both children and adults, often accompanied by significant sleep disturbances. Recent studies, including longitudinal research and experimental sleep manipulation, have confirmed a strong association between short sleep duration, typically defined as 6 hours or less per night, and an increase in ADHD symptoms, particularly inattention and oppositional behaviors. In contrast, long sleep duration does not appear to have a significant correlation with ADHD, highlighting the importance of sleep restriction rather than excessive sleep as a key factor in the disorder's symptomatology. Various neurobiological mechanisms contribute to this relationship, including disruptions in circadian rhythms, alterations in the dopaminergic system, increased physiological and cognitive hyperarousal, and deficits in executive functioning. These mechanisms collectively impair sleep regulation and exacerbate the difficulties in maintaining healthy sleep patterns among individuals with ADHD. This chapter explores the complex bidirectional link between ADHD and sleep disturbances, discussing diagnostic challenges, effective therapeutic interventions, and directions for future research that may lead to more personalized treatment strategies.

Keywords: ADHD, sleep disorders, insomnia, circadian rhythm, restless legs syndrome, polysomnography, melatonin, neurodevelopment

1. Introduction

Attention-Deficit/Hyperactivity Disorder (ADHD) is a prevalent neurodevelopmental condition that affects children, adolescents, and adults worldwide. Characterized by persistent patterns of inattention, hyperactivity, and impulsivity, ADHD significantly impacts daily functioning, academic performance, and overall well-being. While ADHD is traditionally understood in the context of cognitive and behavioral impairments, a growing body of research highlights the critical role of sleep disturbances in the disorder's symptomatology. Individuals with ADHD frequently experience difficulties with sleep onset, maintenance, and quality, leading to chronic sleep deprivation that exacerbates attention deficits, emotional dysregulation, and executive dysfunction [1, 2].

The relationship between ADHD and sleep disorders is complex and bidirectional. On one hand, the neurobiological mechanisms underlying ADHD—such as dopaminergic pathway dysfunction (particularly involving the mesocorticolimbic and nigrostriatal circuits) [3], alterations in circadian rhythms [4] and increased physiological arousal—directly contribute to disrupted sleep patterns. On the other hand, inadequate or poor-quality sleep further worsens ADHD symptoms, creating a vicious cycle in which cognitive and behavioral impairments are perpetuated by chronic sleep deficits. Dopamine plays a crucial role in modulating both arousal and REM/NREM sleep transitions [5], and its imbalance contributes to the instability of the sleep-wake cycle observed in ADHD. Despite increasing recognition of this connection, sleep disturbances remain an often-overlooked aspect of ADHD diagnosis and treatment.

Given the strong interplay between sleep and ADHD, understanding the mechanisms linking the two is essential for improving therapeutic interventions. This chapter explores the neurobiological underpinnings of sleep dysfunction in ADHD, examines the specific sleep disorders commonly associated with the condition, and discusses diagnostic challenges and treatment strategies. Additionally, it highlights the importance of personalized approaches to managing sleep problems in individuals with ADHD and outlines key directions for future research. By addressing the sleep-related aspects of ADHD, clinicians and researchers can develop more comprehensive treatment plans that not only target core ADHD symptoms but also improve overall sleep health and quality of life. An illustrative figure summarizing the interaction between dopaminergic pathways, sleep regulation, and ADHD symptoms would further enhance clarity for the reader.

2. Neurobiological mechanisms

Sleep disturbances in ADHD can be attributed to multiple neurobiological factors. One of the most prominent is dopaminergic dysfunction, with alterations in the dopamine transporter (DAT) and receptors (D1/D2) affecting arousal regulation, reward sensitivity, and sleep-wake stability [3]. The mesolimbic dopamine pathway (ventral tegmental area–nucleus accumbens) and the nigrostriatal pathway (substantia nigra–striatum) are both implicated in ADHD and play key roles in sleep initiation and REM regulation. Research has demonstrated that individuals with ADHD often present with polymorphisms in the dopamine transporter gene (DAT1), which affects arousal levels and contributes to instability in REM sleep [6]. Additionally, circadian rhythm dysregulation plays a critical role, as many individuals with ADHD exhibit a delayed sleep phase, characterized by later sleep onset, shorter overall sleep duration, and increased daytime sleepiness. These disruptions are often linked to alterations in melatonin secretion, mutations in clock genes, and a strong preference for evening activities, which further misaligns their sleep patterns with conventional social and academic schedules [7].

Another key factor is the imbalance in arousal levels. Individuals with ADHD frequently experience hyperarousal, making it difficult to transition into sleep. This heightened state of alertness is associated with increased autonomic nervous system activity and altered cortical excitability, which leads to fragmented sleep, frequent nocturnal awakenings, and reduced sleep efficiency. Additionally, research indicates that adolescents with ADHD exhibit greater intraindividual variability in their sleep-wake patterns, meaning that their sleep duration and quality fluctuate significantly from night to night. Such irregularity may be linked to dopaminergic instability within the striatal-prefrontal circuits, influencing both sleep quality and executive

DOI: http://dx.doi.org/10.5772/intechopen.1012709

function [8]. This irregularity in sleep patterns can negatively impact cognitive performance and emotional regulation, further exacerbating the core symptoms of ADHD (**Figure 1**) [9].

2.1 The relationship between ADHD and specific sleep disorders

ADHD is frequently associated with several distinct sleep disorders, each of which contributes to the overall burden of symptoms. Insomnia is among the most common, with individuals reporting persistent difficulties in initiating and maintaining sleep. This often stems from emotional dysregulation, increased nighttime activity, and racing thoughts, which prevent relaxation before bedtime. In addition to insomnia, restless legs syndrome (RLS) is also highly prevalent among individuals with ADHD, largely due to underlying dopaminergic dysfunction. This condition is characterized by an uncomfortable urge to move the legs, particularly at night, leading to sleep fragmentation and excessive daytime sleepiness [10, 11].

Another sleep disorder frequently observed in ADHD is obstructive sleep apnea (OSA), a condition marked by snoring, repeated pauses in breathing, and daytime fatigue. The symptoms of OSA can mimic those of ADHD, such as inattentiveness and hyperactivity, making accurate diagnosis particularly challenging. Similarly, delayed sleep phase syndrome (DSPS) is another common sleep disturbance, in which individuals experience a significant misalignment of their circadian rhythms [12]. Those with ADHD often struggle with late sleep onset and difficulty waking in the morning, leading to chronic sleep deprivation and impaired cognitive functioning during the day. Periodic limb movement disorder (PLMD) is yet another condition frequently co-occurring with ADHD, involving involuntary limb movements during sleep that result in frequent nighttime awakenings and daytime inattention. Each of these sleep disorders can independently contribute to the worsening of ADHD symptoms, underscoring the need for thorough sleep assessments in individuals diagnosed with the condition [13].

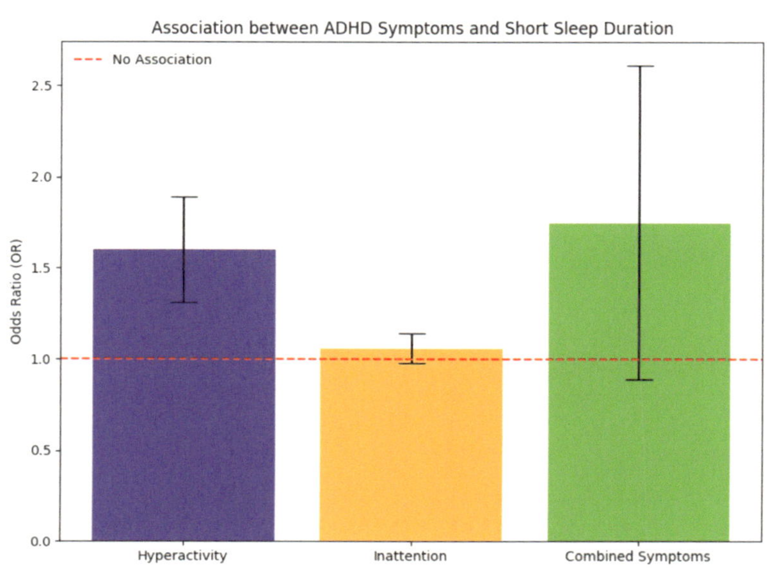

Figure 1.
Neurobiological mechanisms linking dopaminergic dysfunction, circadian rhythm disruption, and sleep-wake instability in ADHD. Source: Figure from [3].

2.2 The impact of reduced sleep duration on ADHD symptoms

The provided graph illustrates the relationship between ADHD symptoms and reduced sleep duration, based on a systematic review and meta-analysis of observational studies [14]. Additional studies have reinforced that chronic sleep restriction worsens hyperactivity, inattention, and emotional dysregulation in ADHD patients (**Figure 2**).

The main findings of the review indicate:

- Hyperactivity: This symptom is significantly associated with reduced sleep duration, with an odds ratio (OR) of 1.60 (95% confidence interval: 1.18–2.17). This suggests that individuals who get less sleep are more likely to exhibit hyperactivity compared to the average sleep duration.

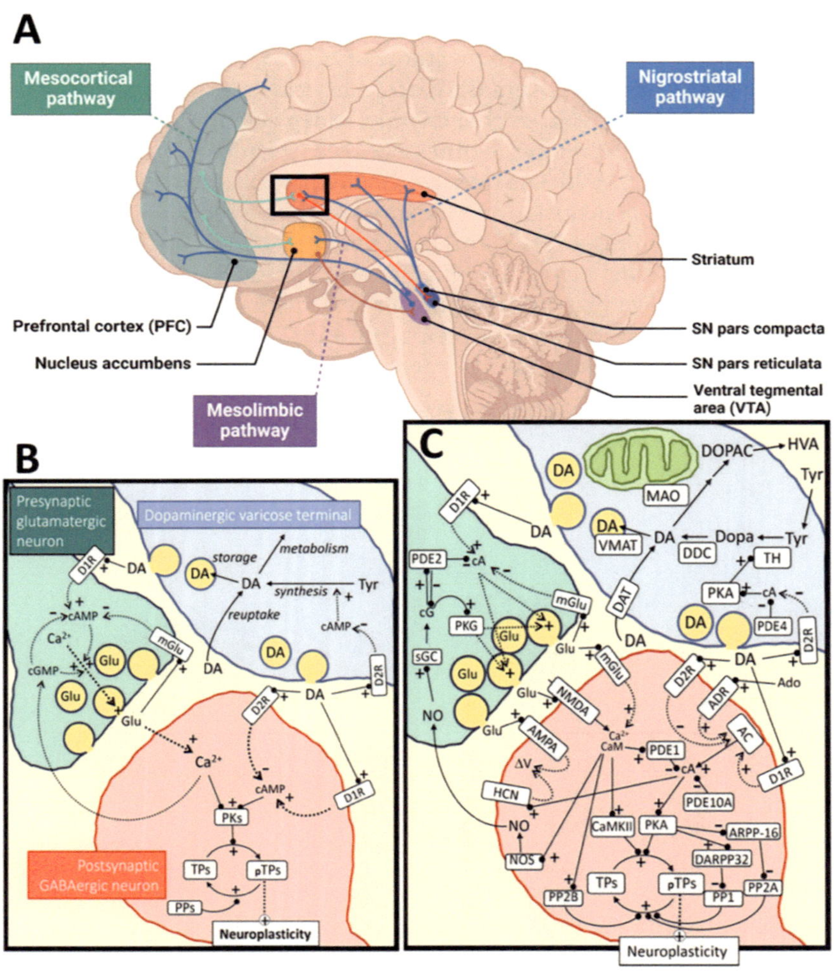

Figure 2.
Association between reduced sleep duration and ADHD symptoms, highlighting differential effects on hyperactivity and inattention.

- Inattention: This symptom shows a weaker association with reduced sleep duration, with an OR close to 1, indicating a less pronounced or potentially non-significant relationship.

- Combined symptoms (hyperactivity and inattention): These present an overall association with reduced sleep duration but with greater variability (wide confidence interval), suggesting that the results may be influenced by other factors.

3. Diagnostic considerations

Given the significant overlap between ADHD and sleep disturbances, a comprehensive and multidimensional assessment approach is necessary to differentiate primary ADHD symptoms from those arising because of sleep disorders. Clinical history and standardized sleep questionnaires are essential tools in this process. Instruments such as the Children's Sleep Habits Questionnaire (CSHQ), the Pittsburgh Sleep Quality Index (PSQI), and the Epworth Sleepiness Scale (ESS) help clinicians evaluate the severity and nature of sleep problems [15]. Additionally, objective sleep assessments provide further insights into sleep patterns. Polysomnography, for instance, is particularly useful in identifying structural abnormalities in sleep architecture, diagnosing conditions such as OSA and PLMD, and assessing REM sleep stability. Similarly, actigraphy, which involves the continuous monitoring of movement patterns, is a valuable tool for detecting circadian rhythm disruptions and variability in sleep duration. Furthermore, the multiple sleep latency test (MSLT) is often employed to assess excessive daytime sleepiness, a symptom that is particularly relevant for individuals with ADHD who struggle with sustained attention and alertness. In cases where delayed sleep phase syndrome is suspected, melatonin secretion analysis can be conducted to determine whether melatonin onset is significantly delayed, providing additional confirmation of circadian misalignment [16].

4. Treatment and management strategies

Effectively managing sleep disturbances in ADHD requires a multimodal approach that integrates behavioral, pharmacological, and chronotherapeutic interventions. Behavioral interventions, particularly sleep hygiene education, play a foundational role in improving sleep quality [17]. Establishing a consistent bedtime routine, reducing screen exposure in the evening, and limiting the intake of stimulants such as caffeine have been shown to significantly improve sleep outcomes. Additionally, cognitive behavioral therapy for insomnia (CBT-I) has emerged as an effective intervention for addressing sleep-onset difficulties in ADHD, helping individuals develop healthier sleep associations and relaxation techniques [18].

Pharmacological treatments are also frequently utilized to address ADHD-related sleep disturbances. Melatonin supplementation, particularly in low doses ranging from 0.5 to 5 mg, has been found to be beneficial for individuals experiencing circadian misalignment, helping to regulate sleep onset and improve sleep duration. For individuals with ADHD who also suffer from restless legs syndrome, iron supplementation may be recommended, especially in cases where ferritin levels are low. In addition, alpha-2 adrenergic agonists such as clonidine and guanfacine have been shown to facilitate sleep initiation and reduce nighttime awakenings. Adjustments in stimulant medication timing may also be necessary, as stimulant use too close to bedtime can exacerbate sleep difficulties [19].

Chronotherapy, which focuses on adjusting the body's internal clock, is another promising avenue for treatment. Bright light therapy, for example, has been demonstrated to effectively reset circadian rhythms in individuals with delayed sleep phase syndrome, gradually shifting sleep onset to an earlier time. Similarly, a structured approach to sleep phase advancement, in which bedtime is progressively adjusted earlier, can help realign sleep cycles with societal norms [20].

5. Future research directions

Future studies should focus on identifying genetic markers that predict which individuals with ADHD are most likely to develop sleep disturbances. Additionally, neuroimaging studies may provide deeper insights into the structural and functional brain changes associated with both ADHD and sleep disorders [21, 22]. Longitudinal research examining sleep patterns across different developmental stages could shed light on how sleep disturbances evolve from childhood to adulthood in individuals with ADHD. Furthermore, alternative therapeutic approaches, such as cannabidiol (CBD), digital therapeutics, and mindfulness-based interventions, should be explored as potential non-pharmacological treatments for improving sleep quality. More research is also needed to assess the long-term effects of stimulant and non-stimulant medications on sleep architecture, as this remains an area of significant clinical concern [23].

6. Conclusion

The interplay between ADHD and sleep disturbances is complex and multifaceted, with short sleep duration emerging as a particularly influential factor in worsening ADHD symptoms [18]. The neurobiological underpinnings of this relationship, including dopaminergic dysfunction, circadian misalignment, and hyperarousal, highlight the need for targeted interventions that address both sleep and ADHD symptoms concurrently. Early diagnosis and tailored interventions, including melatonin therapy, behavioral modifications, and sleep hygiene education, are essential for optimizing sleep quality and improving ADHD symptom control. As research in this field continues to evolve, a more personalized approach to treatment may ultimately enhance the well-being of individuals affected by both ADHD and sleep disorders.

Acknowledgements

The author(s) acknowledge the use of the AI tool ChatGPT (OpenAI, San Francisco, CA, USA) exclusively for language editing purposes in the preparation of this manuscript.

Conflict of interest

The authors declare that they have no conflicts of interest.

Author details

Martina Gnazzo[1,4], Valentina Baldini[1,2], Giulia Santangelo[3], Giuditta Bargiacchi[4] and Marco Carotenuto[4*]

1 Department of Biomedical, Metabolic and Neural Sciences, University of Modena and Reggio Emilia, Italy

2 Department of Biomedical and Neuromotor Sciences, University of Bologna, Italy

3 Department of Health Sciences, University of Milan, Milan, Italy

4 Sleep Lab for Developmental Age, Clinic of Child and Adolescent Neuropsychiatry, Department of Mental Health, Physical and Preventive Medicine, University of Campania "Luigi Vanvitelli", Italy

*Address all correspondence to: marco.carotenuto@unicampania.it

References

[1] Becker SP, Epstein JN, Tamm L, Tilford AA, Tischner CM, Isaacson PA, et al. Shortened sleep duration causes sleepiness, inattention, and oppositionality in adolescents with ADHD: Findings from a crossover sleep restriction/extension study. Journal of the American Academy of Child and Adolescent Psychiatry. 2019;**58**(4):433-442

[2] Carpena MX, Munhoz TN, Xavier MO, Rohde LA, Santos IS, Del-Ponte B, et al. The role of sleep duration and sleep problems during childhood in the development of ADHD in adolescence: Findings from a population-based birth cohort. Journal of Attention Disorders. 2020;**24**(4):590-600

[3] MacDonald HJ, Kleppe R, Szigetvari PD, Haavik J. The dopamine hypothesis for ADHD: An evaluation of evidence accumulated from human studies and animal models. Frontiers in Psychiatry. 2024;**15**:1492126. DOI: 10.3389/fpsyt.2024.1492126

[4] van Andel E, Bijlenga D, Vogel SWN, Beekman ATF, Kooij JJS. Attention-deficit/hyperactivity disorder and delayed sleep phase syndrome in adults: A randomized clinical trial on the effects of chronotherapy on sleep. Journal of Biological Rhythms. 2022;**37**(6):673-689. DOI: 10.1177/07487304221124659. Epub 2022 Sep 30

[5] Eban-Rothschild A, Appelbaum L, de Lecea L. Neuronal mechanisms for sleep/wake regulation and modulatory drive. Neuropsychopharmacology. 2018;**43**(5):937-952. DOI: 10.1038/npp.2017.294. Epub 2017 Dec 5

[6] Lam LT, Yang L. Duration of sleep and ADHD tendency among adolescents in China. Journal of Attention Disorders. 2008;**11**(4):437-444

[7] Wajszilber D, Santiseban JA, Gruber R. Sleep disorders in patients with ADHD: Impact and management challenges. Nature and Science of Sleep. 2018;**10**:453-480

[8] Langberg JM, Breaux RP, Cusick CN, Green CD, Smith ZR, Molitor SJ, et al. Intraindividual variability of sleep/wake patterns in adolescents with and without attention-deficit/hyperactivity disorder. Journal of Child Psychology and Psychiatry. 2019;**60**(11):1219-1229. DOI: 10.1111/jcpp.13082. Epub 2019 Jun 24

[9] Van Veen MM, Kooij JJS, Boonstra AM, Gordijn MCM, Van Someren EJW. Delayed circadian rhythm in adults with ADHD. Biological Psychiatry. 2010;**67**(11):1091-1096

[10] Langberg JM, Breaux RP, Cusick CN, Green CD, Smith ZR, Molitor SJ, et al. Intraindividual variability of sleep/wake patterns in adolescents with and without ADHD. Journal of Child Psychology and Psychiatry. 2019;**60**(11):1219-1229

[11] Tong L, Ye Y, Yan Q. The moderating roles of bedtime activities and anxiety/depression in the relationship between attention-deficit/hyperactivity disorder symptoms and sleep problems in children. BMC Psychiatry. 2018;**18**:298

[12] Hiscock H, Sciberras E, editors. Sleep and ADHD: An Evidence-Based Guide to Assessment and Treatment San Diego. CA: Elsevier/Academic Press; 2019

[13] Lee SH, Kim HB, Lee KW. Association between sleep duration and attention-deficit hyperactivity disorder: A systematic review and meta-analysis

of observational studies. Journal of Affective Disorders. 2019;**256**:62-69. DOI: 10.1016/j.jad.2019.05.071. Epub 2019 May 28

[14] Cortese S, Faraone SV, Konofal E, Lecendreux M. Sleep in children with attention-deficit/hyperactivity disorder: Meta-analysis of subjective and objective studies. Journal of the American Academy of Child and Adolescent Psychiatry. 2009;**48**:894-908

[15] Crowley SJ, Wolfson AR, Tarokh L, Carskadon MA. An update on adolescent sleep: New evidence informing the perfect storm model. Journal of Adolescence. 2018;**67**:55-65

[16] Lunsford-Avery JR, Krystal AD, Kollins SH. Sleep disturbances in adolescents with ADHD: A systematic review and framework for future research. Clinical Psychology Review. 2016;**50**:159-174

[17] Bourchtein E, Langberg JM, Cusick CN, Breaux RP, Smith ZR, Becker SP. Technology use and sleep in adolescents with and without attention-deficit/hyperactivity disorder. Journal of Pediatric Psychology. 2019;**44**:517-526

[18] Martin CA, Hiscock H, Rinehart N, Heussler HS, Hyde C, Fuller-Tyszkiewicz M, et al. Associations between sleep hygiene and sleep problems in adolescents with ADHD: A cross-sectional study. Journal of Attention Disorders. Feb 2020;**24**(4):545-554. DOI: 10.1177/1087054718762513. Epub 2018 Mar 15. PMID: 29542374

[19] Meltzer LJ. Future directions in sleep and developmental psychopathology. Journal of Clinical Child and Adolescent Psychology. 2017;**46**:295-301

[20] Landau R, Sadeh A, Vassoly P, Berger A, Atzaba-Poria N, Auerbach JG. Sleep patterns of 7-week-old infants at familial risk for attention deficit hyperactivity disorder. Infant Mental Health Journal. 2010;**31**:630-646

[21] Dahl RE. The regulation of sleep and arousal: Development and psychopathology. Development and Psychopathology. 1996;**8**:3-27

[22] Gruber R, Wiebe S, Montecalvo L, Brunetti B, Amsel R, Carrier J. Impact of sleep restriction on neurobehavioral functioning of children with attention deficit hyperactivity disorder. Sleep. 2011;**34**:315-323

[23] Cremone-Caira A, Root H, Harvey EA, McDermott JM, Spencer RMC. Effects of sleep extension on inhibitory control in children with ADHD: A pilot study. Journal of Attention Disorders. Feb 2020;**24**(4):601-610. DOI: 10.1177/1087054719851575. Epub 2019 May 29. PMID: 31138037; PMCID: PMC7887756

Section 2

Innovation and Translational Pathways in ADHD Diagnosis and Care

Chapter 5

ADHD Co-Occurring Conditions: A Multidisciplinary Approach

Jamuna Das and Jitendriya Biswal

Abstract

Attention-deficit/hyperactivity disorder (ADHD) rarely manifests itself in isolation as a straightforward clinical syndrome but rather occurs in a mixture of clinically relevant neurodevelopmental, psychiatric, and somatic comorbidities. The heterogeneous manifestation of phenotypic forms highlights the interdisciplinarity of the methods involved, necessitating an integrated approach that draws from medical, psychological, educational, and sociocultural perspectives. It is this view of heterogeneity, or evidence of variability in clinical features of ADHD, that this chapter reflects upon. This chapter is primarily concerned with evidence-based interventions that facilitate the adoption of integrative diagnostic approaches and the implementation of multimodal treatment models. In the spirit of interdisciplinarity as well as individualized treatment models, this chapter aims to support a systems-based approach to ADHD that focuses on the maximization of function beyond symptom management and long-term adaptation. It supports integrated models of the multifactorial etiology of ADHD, as well as the psychosocial burden across the lifespan, while acknowledging the relevance of functional outcome assessment.

Keywords: ADHD, comorbidity, multidisciplinary care, mental health disorders, neurodevelopmental conditions, integrated treatment

1. Introduction

ADHD frequently co-occurs with other conditions, such as anxiety disorders, depression, autism spectrum disorder (ASD), learning disabilities, oppositional defiant disorder (ODD), and substance use disorders (SUDs). The presence of these comorbid conditions makes the presentation of ADHD more difficult to diagnose and treat [1, 2]. The likelihood of comorbid ADHD implies a shared genetic and neurobiological basis for other psychiatric and developmental disorders. Research has shown that individuals with ADHD have a significantly increased risk of developing other behavioural disorders, as well as mood and anxiety disorders, compared to the general population [3]. The comorbidity of symptoms can lead to underdiagnosis or misdiagnosis, potentially postponing interventions that could improve quality of life. For instance, a child with affective anxiety and ADHD may have difficulties with inattention, yet the underlying cause of his or her difficulties, whether due to affective anxiety or ADHD symptoms, is difficult to disentangle. Such diagnostic intricacy works to affirm the necessity for intensive assessments to consider the broader mental health profile of individuals who have ADHD [3, 4].

Anxiety disorders are the most frequent co-occurring disorders among patients with ADHD. According to studies, 50% or more of those with ADHD report considerable anxiety symptoms [3]. Anxiety has a way of exacerbating impairments associated with ADHD, such as problems with concentration and completing tasks, by layering over it an element of emotional distress [5, 6]. Similarly, depression also commonly co-occurs with ADHD, and studies have shown that children and adults with ADHD are more at risk of developing major depressive disorder than those without ADHD [7]. The combination of ADHD and depression can be especially troubling, as ADHD's difficulties with executive functioning, impulsivity, and social issues can lead to feelings of frustration, self-worth issues, and hopelessness [8].

Autism spectrum disorder (ASD) also often occurs together with ADHD, with estimates by studies indicating that 30–50% of those with ASD have symptoms of ADHD. Although ADHD and ASD are two different conditions, they have similar features, like impaired impulse control, social interactions, and executive function [9]. The co-occurrence of the two disorders in a single person makes it challenging to treat since interventions for one disorder might not be fully effective for the other. Furthermore, learning disabilities impact an estimated 30–50% of the ADHD population [10], adding further problems in school and workplace environments. Students with ADHD and learning disabilities are frequently poor readers, writers, or mathematicians, which can result in frustration, reduced academic functioning, and higher rates of school dropout [11, 12].

Oppositional defiant disorder (ODD) is another common co-occurring condition, particularly in children with ADHD. ODD is characterized by persistent patterns of defiant, disobedient, and hostile behavior toward authority figures [13]. The impulsivity and emotional dysregulation associated with ADHD can exacerbate ODD symptoms, leading to difficulties in family, school, and social environments. If left unaddressed, ODD can progress into more severe conduct disorders (CDs) in adolescence and adulthood, further complicating long-term outcomes [14, 15].

Substance abuse disorders are also substantially more common among people with ADHD, especially in teenagers and adults. Individuals with ADHD have been found by studies to have an elevated risk of early drug use, addiction, and a more severe course of drug use. The risk-taking and impulsive nature of ADHD can also be responsible for the higher likelihood of using substances as a method of coping. Additionally, undiagnosed ADHD symptoms, especially those of emotional dysregulation and executive dysfunction, can cause individuals to self-medicate with alcohol, nicotine, or illegal drugs [16, 17].

ADHD is a complex condition, especially when it comes with other issues, so a multidisciplinary approach to both diagnosis and treatment is key. Clinicians should adopt a thorough assessment strategy that looks at the entire range of symptoms and helps to differentiate between overlapping conditions. Treatment plans need to be personalized to address both ADHD and any coexisting disorders, using a blend of behavioral interventions, psychoeducation, medication, and therapy. For example, stimulant medications like methylphenidate and amphetamines are frequently used for ADHD, but it is important to monitor their impact on any anxiety or mood disorders that might also be present. Cognitive behavioral therapy (CBT), social skills training, and parent training programs can also play a significant role in effectively managing ADHD and its associated conditions.

1.1 Understanding ADHD co-occurring conditions

These conditions include anxiety disorders, depression, learning disabilities, oppositional defiant disorder, and substance use disorders, to name a few. It is important to understand the connection between ADHD and these co-occurring conditions, as doing so allows for correct diagnosis, effective treatment, and comprehensive care. This section will delve into the more commonly discussed comorbidities, in what ways they might exacerbate ADHD symptoms, and what these comorbidities look like at different ages and points in life [18]. ADHD often conjures images of children with inattentive or hyperactive behaviors; however, symptoms can manifest and persist into adulthood. Adult ADHD is complex in its own right, but additional complexity arises frequently in the form of co-occurring (or comorbid) conditions, i.e., mental health conditions or physical health complications that co-occur with an ADHD diagnosis (**Figure 1**).

1.2 Anxiety disorders

Multiple adults and children with attention-deficit/hyperactivity disorder (ADHD) have comorbid anxiety disorders, such as generalized anxiety disorder (GAD), social anxiety disorder, and panic disorder. Anxiety can amplify ADHD symptoms as well as impact emotional regulation and executive functioning. It is also appreciated that comorbid anxiety disorders occur frequently in children diagnosed with ADHD; this may affect 25–50% of children diagnosed with ADHD [19, 20]. ADHD and anxiety disorders are frequent comorbid conditions, but the contributory risk factors of ADHD and anxiety disorders are still poorly understood [19, 21, 22]. By examining how these factors interact across different stages of development, researchers can identify early indicators of risk and resilience. This perspective also highlights the importance of studying the role of family dynamics, peer relationships, genetic predispositions, and neurobiological mechanisms in shaping the trajectories of adult ADHD and anxiety [23, 24].

Developmental psychopathology emphasizes the convergence of typical and atypical developmental processes and allows for a more fulfilling explanation of the development and course of mental health disorders. For example, children with ADHD have challenges

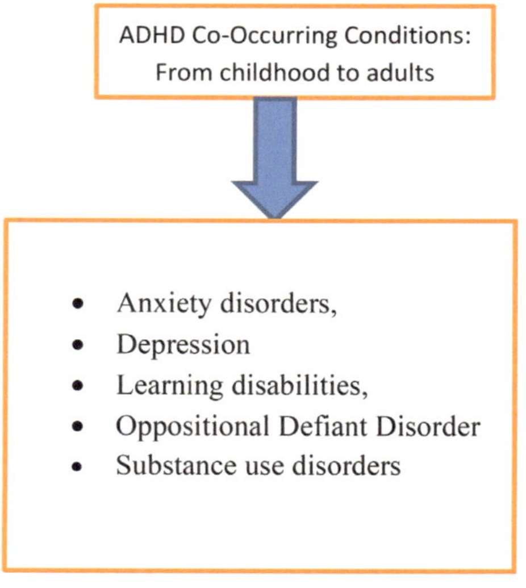

Figure 1.
Common co-occurring conditions associated with Attention-Deficit/Hyperactivity Disorder (ADHD) across the lifespan include anxiety disorders, depression, learning disabilities, Oppositional Defiant Disorder, and substance use disorders.

with emotional regulation and executive functioning that can predispose them to anxiety. Chronic stressors, such as family conflict, academic difficulties, or problems with peers, all increase both ADHD and anxiety symptoms [25, 26]. Biological causes, such as genetic predisposition and neurobiological abnormalities, also have an important role. Genetic susceptibility could help to explain why the disorders co-occur. Abnormalities in brain areas that play roles in attention, emotion regulation, and stress response, the prefrontal cortex and amygdala, are frequently implicated [27, 28]. Social and environmental factors further influence the risk for anxiety and ADHD. Parenting style, socioeconomic status, and trauma exposure can have long-lasting effects on the child's mental health. Interventions and supportive family environments can counteract these risks, highlighting the need for early identification and targeted interventions [29, 30].

Future research that taps into longitudinal studies and cutting-edge neuroimaging techniques can really deepen our understanding of how ADHD and anxiety develop over time. It is crucial to take a comprehensive, multidisciplinary approach that looks at the intricate interplay between biological, social, and psychological factors. This way, we can create effective prevention and intervention strategies. By adopting a developmental psychopathology perspective, clinicians and researchers can more accurately spot children who are at risk and offer personalized support to foster positive developmental outcomes.

2. Depression

Among the most common and impactful of these co-occurring disorders is depression. From childhood through adulthood, individuals with ADHD face an increased risk of experiencing depressive symptoms, which can complicate diagnosis, treatment, and daily functioning. Understanding the intricate relationship between ADHD and depression is essential not only for effective clinical management but also for fostering awareness, empathy, and support for those affected. This introduction sets the stage for exploring how these conditions interact over time, shaping emotional development and mental health across the lifespan [31]. When depression co-occurs with adult ADHD, symptoms may overlap or worsen. Depression can lead to low mood, lack of motivation, and difficulty concentrating, symptoms that can be mistaken for or compounded by ADHD. This overlap makes diagnosis and treatment more complex [32].

When diagnosing ADHD with co-occurring depression from childhood into adulthood, it is essential to consider the overlapping and compounding effects of both conditions. ADHD may present as inattention, impulsivity, and emotional dysregulation, while co-occurring depression often manifests as persistent sadness, low energy, and negative self-perception—symptoms that can be mistaken for or worsened by untreated ADHD. A thorough evaluation should include clinical interviews, behavior checklists, and developmental history. Treatment typically involves a multimodal approach: stimulant or non-stimulant medications to manage ADHD symptoms, combined with cognitive behavioral therapy (CBT) to address depressive thoughts and develop executive functioning skills. Ongoing psychoeducation and family support are crucial in promoting long-term coping strategies and functional well-being [33–40].

3. Mood disorders

Mood conditions, including bipolar disorder and depression, tend to co-occur with ADHD in adults, in particular [41]. Chronic stress and frustration, stemming from ADHD's difficulties, can heighten the risk of developing a mood disorder. In addition, both genetic and environmental sources are responsible for this comorbidity. Diagnosis proves complicated, as depressive periods or manic states in bipolar disorder may masquerade as ADHD symptomology [41]. The comorbidity of ADHD and mood conditions is rooted deeply in the brain's complex circuitry. Both conditions are linked with dopamine and norepinephrine imbalances, chemical secretions that control mood, motivation, and attention. Genetic predispositions also play an influential part, with family histories of ADHD or bipolar disorder raising the chances of their co-occurrence [42, 43]. Environmental sources of stress, along with lifetime challenges, also contribute to heightening symptoms. Battling with unmapped ADHD symptoms, such as forgetfulness or impulsiveness, may result in feelings of frustration and criticism, serving as fertile ground for developing depressive ideation. Moreover, the unpredictable cycles of bipolar disorder's mood swings may enhance ADHD's difficulties, with stability proving elusive in maintaining this complicated interplay of conditions [44].

Emotion regulation is yet another link that ties all of these conditions together. While emotional impulsivity is commonly linked with ADHD, mood disorders may result in pervasive sadness, hopelessness, or irritability [45]. For instance, an individual with both ADHD and depression may feel extremely tired and unmotivated, unable to get even simple activities done. Conversely, the manic episode in bipolar disorder can increase impulsivity, leading to impulsive decision-making and excessive self-confidence [46]. Because of the convergent symptoms, it is challenging for clinicians to differentiate in which condition ADHD stops and a mood disorder begins, highlighting the need for a careful and detailed diagnostic process. Luckily, treatment methods are in place that can treat the intricacy of comorbid ADHD and mood disorders [43, 47]. Many times, medications, for instance, the use of stimulants in the case of ADHD and mood stabilizers or antidepressants for the treatment of mood disorders, are administered together to manage the symptoms. Psychotherapy, especially cognitive behavioral therapy (CBT), also offers significant means for individuals to manage their emotions [48]. Sessions of therapy can promote coping techniques that treat both the difficulty of attention as well as the instability of moods. Lifestyle changes, in the form of regular exercise, regular sleep, and practices of being mindful, usually go a long way in emotional and cognitive welfare [49]. Treating both conditions together, individuals usually get in command of themselves and develop resilience. Living with both ADHD and a mood disorder is indisputably challenging, but it also provides avenues for personal growth and insight.

4. Learning disabilities

This study shows that ADHD commonly co-occurs with other learning disabilities, such as dyslexia, dyscalculia, and specific learning disabilities (SLDs). Comorbidity can create challenges in diagnosing and treating ADHD and can introduce additional barriers in school and social contexts. Knowledge about the relationship between learning disabilities and ADHD is essential when designing educational treatment.

Dyslexia: Margaret et al. conducted a study about dyslexia: past, present, and future. Dyslexia is one of the most common learning disabilities, which involves difficulty with reading, decoding words, and spelling despite appropriate intelligence and instruction. Studies show that 20–30% of children with ADHD also have dyslexia [50]. When children have both of these conditions, it creates a unique set of difficulties for them, as the reading and attention problems may impact each other.

Dyscalculia: Haberstroh and Schulte-Körne present a review of research on the diagnosis and treatment of dyscalculia, offering insights into current diagnostic criteria, intervention strategies, and the effectiveness of various therapeutic approaches. Dyscalculia is a specific learning disability that affects people's understanding of numbers, calculation, and solving math problems. Dyscalculia, just like dyslexia, can co-occur with ADHD. It is estimated that as many as 30% of children with ADHD also have reading and spelling disorders [51]. Children with ADHD often experience difficulties regulating their attention and memory, which can compound the challenges associated with understanding concepts like mathematical anxiety and school phobia, creating a seemingly untenable cycle of frustration and academic underachievement.

Other specific learning disabilities (SLDs) that also occur in childhood are reading, writing, and math difficulties. Comorbidity of ADHD and SLD has been shown in research, with comorbidity rates of 31–45%. While ADHD is mostly a disorder of behavior with impulsivity and opposition in children, the academic struggles of children with ADHD are usually given little attention. This review emphasizes increased acknowledgment of the learning difficulties inherent in children with ADHD, with a focus on both the treatment of behavior and academic achievement for their overall success and growth [51].

The concurrent presence of ADHD and learning disabilities, including dyslexia, dyscalculia, and other specific learning difficulties, poses special challenges for students in both academic and social environments. They can impede achievement in school and erode a child's sense of self-worth. Yet, with individually focused intervention aimed specifically at attention deficit and learning difficulties, students can dramatically enhance their academic achievement and emotional health. By taking a comprehensive, individualized perspective that includes differentiated instruction, behavioristic approaches, and emotional support, students with ADHD and learning disabilities can be helped by parents and educators to fulfill their potential [52, 53].

5. Oppositional defiant disorder (ODD) and conduct disorder (CD)

Systematic reviews of research consistently show that ADHD, ODD, and CD development and relationships are driven by a complex interaction of genetic and environmental risk factors. While genetics appears to be central to triggering the onset of these disorders, environmental context fundamentally governs the trajectory and outcome of these disorders. Children with ADHD are at an increased risk of developing ODD and CD. Effective early intervention is important, not just for ADHD, but for preventing the subsequent potential development of ODD and CD [54]. These conditions are associated with defiance, aggression, and persistent rule-breaking behavior, often complicating the management of ADHD and significantly impacting the child's development and family life [55].

Oppositional defiant disorder (ODD) is defined as a pattern of angry or irritable mood, argumentative or defiant behavior, and vindictiveness toward an authority figure [56]. Conduct disorder (CD) is typically considered more severe, and symptoms include behaviors that are not in keeping with societal norms and violate the rights of others (e.g., aggression to people and animals, destruction of property, deceitfulness, serious violations of rules) [57]. These statistics stress the necessity for early diagnosis and comprehensive intervention strategies.

There are several reasons children with ADHD face an increased risk for ODD and CD:

1. Neurological and genetic similarities: There are several established genetic and neurobiological risk factors that ADHD, ODD, and CD share; perhaps most strikingly, they often share some dysfunction in the prefrontal cortex, which regulates decision-making and impulse control [58, 59].

   a. Environmental influences: Children with ADHD may experience frequent negative interactions with parents, teachers, and peers due to their impulsive or disruptive behaviors. This can create a cycle of conflict and punishment that fosters defiance and resentment [54].

   b. Poor emotional regulation: ADHD is often associated with difficulties in managing emotions, which can escalate into the more confrontational behaviors seen in ODD and CD if not appropriately addressed [15].

Effective management of comorbid ADHD and behavioral disorders involves a multimodal approach, with a particular focus on behavioral therapy and structured environments.

1. Behavioral therapy: Cognitive behavioral therapy (CBT) and parent management training are evidence-based interventions that teach children and caregivers how to manage behaviors, set appropriate limits, and reinforce positive behavior [60, 61].

2. Structured environments: The growth of children can be facilitated, and behavioral disruptions can be significantly reduced by creating consistent routines, clear expectations, and organized activities. Schools and households using positive behavioral support systems realize more favorable results for children with ADHD and behavior disorders [60, 62].

3. Medication: While stimulant medications are commonly used to manage ADHD symptoms, they are often insufficient in treating ODD or CD on their own. However, when combined with therapy, medication can play a supportive role [63, 64].

6. Autism spectrum disorder (ASD)

Autism spectrum disorder (ASD) and ADHD are two unique disorders that stem from a person's neurodevelopmental system. Each has its defining characteristics and criteria for diagnosis [65]. Nevertheless, there has been growing research on the overlap of these disorders, especially with the common symptoms and core brain structures. Those with co-occurring ADHD and ASD face all the heightened challenges of both and require specialized, integrated approaches to interventions that have multifaceted approaches to treatment [65, 66].

ASD is characterized by persistent social communication and interaction deficits, together with limited, repetitive behavioral patterns. Despite their differences, both conditions share several overlapping features [66–69]. Children with ASD can exhibit impulsive behaviors and high activity levels similar to those seen in ADHD. These symptoms may manifest as difficulty waiting for turns [9, 70], interrupting conversations, or engaging in physically risky behavior. Social interaction difficulties are common in both conditions. For people with ADHD, social interactions are difficult due to impulsivity, whereas for those with ASD, difficulties come from grasping social cues and reciprocal conversations [70, 71]. Sensory processing issues are a hallmark of ASD but are increasingly recognized in individuals with ADHD as well. Sensory over-responsivity, under-responsivity, or sensory-seeking behaviors may be found in both groups [72].

Multidisciplinary assessment: Comprehensive evaluations by psychologists, psychiatrists, occupational therapists, and speech-language pathologists can help in identifying the full scope of challenges [73, 74].

- Individualized treatment plans: Combining behavioral therapies with pharmacological interventions (where appropriate), tailored to the individual's symptom profile and sensitivities.

- Parental and educational support: Training and support for caregivers and teachers to understand and manage the complexities of dual diagnosis.

- Sensory integration therapies: These are especially beneficial for individuals with heightened sensory sensitivities, which are often present in both disorders.

7. Substance use disorders (SUDs)

While it primarily affects children, its symptoms often continue into adolescence and adulthood. One of the significant concerns associated with ADHD is the increased risk of developing substance use disorders (SUDs) [24, 75]. Research indicates that individuals with ADHD are more likely to misuse substances such as alcohol, nicotine, and illicit drugs. This chapter explores the relationship between ADHD and SUDs, emphasizing the role of impulsivity [24, 75], self-medication tendencies, and the protective impact of early intervention and behavioral therapy.

7.1 ADHD and the risk of substance use disorders

Multiple studies have shown that individuals with ADHD are at a substantially higher risk of developing SUDs compared to the general population. The impulsivity associated with their ADHD can result in kids making poor choices and engaging in risky behaviors; they may also have difficulty engaging in certain behaviors, which may lead to an early drug and alcohol experience, experimentation, or reliance on psychoactive substances [17, 76]. Moreover, many individuals with ADHD may turn to substances as a form of self-medication. They might attempt to alleviate symptoms such as restlessness, distractibility, or emotional dysregulation. Stimulants like nicotine or cocaine may temporarily improve focus and mood, reinforcing substance use behavior [77].

7.2 The role of early intervention

Early identification and treatment of ADHD can significantly reduce the risk of developing SUDs. Behavioral therapy, parent training, and school-based interventions are among the most effective early approaches [78, 79]. When these strategies are implemented in childhood, they can improve emotional regulation, executive functioning, and social skills, which serve as protective factors against later substance use. Pharmacological treatment, particularly with stimulant medications such as methylphenidate or amphetamines, has also been associated with a reduced risk of SUDs when started in childhood and used appropriately [80, 81]. This challenges the earlier concerns that stimulant medication may itself increase the risk of addiction. On the contrary, proper medical management may reduce the likelihood of self-medication and substance misuse later in life.

8. Sleep disorders

Research shows that sleep disturbances are significantly more prevalent in individuals with ADHD compared to the general population. According to Yoon et al. up to 73% of children with ADHD experience some form of sleep problem. In adults, similar trends are reported, with a considerable number experiencing chronic difficulties initiating or maintaining sleep [82]. This bidirectional relationship means that while ADHD can disrupt sleep architecture and circadian rhythms, poor sleep in turn amplifies ADHD symptoms such as forgetfulness, poor emotional regulation, and executive dysfunction. Understanding the mechanisms behind these sleep disorders is essential for effective treatment. Insomnia, characterized by difficulty falling or staying asleep, is the most common sleep disorder among individuals with ADHD [83, 84]. The hyperarousal associated with ADHD, both cognitive and physical, often prevents individuals from relaxing enough to initiate sleep. Additionally, stimulant medications, a primary treatment for ADHD, can interfere with sleep onset if taken too late in the day [85–88]. Behavioral interventions such as adult ADHD cognitive behavioral therapy for insomnia (CBT-I) and mindfulness techniques can be helpful. Adjusting the timing and dosage of medication under medical supervision is also critical [89].

8.1 Restless leg syndrome (RLS)

Restless leg syndrome is another prevalent comorbidity, particularly in children with ADHD. RLS causes uncomfortable sensations in the legs, often described as creeping, crawling, or itching, which are temporarily relieved by movement. This condition is often linked with iron deficiency, which may also contribute to ADHD symptomatology [90]. Assessment of ferritin levels and iron supplementation, if necessary, can improve both RLS and ADHD symptoms. Proper diagnosis is important, as RLS is often underrecognized in pediatric populations [91].

8.2 Delayed sleep phase disorder (DSPD)

Delayed sleep phase disorder is a circadian rhythm disorder characterized by a significant delay in the sleep-wake cycle. Individuals with DSPD feel naturally inclined to fall asleep and wake up much later than societal norms allow [92]. This pattern is commonly seen in adolescents and adults with ADHD [93]. Light therapy, melatonin supplementation, and consistent sleep routines are key interventions. Encouraging natural morning light exposure and limiting screen time in the evening can also be beneficial.

8.3 The role of sleep hygiene

Proper sleep hygiene is foundational in managing sleep issues in ADHD. Key strategies include [94–97]:

- Establishing a consistent bedtime and wake-up schedule
- Creating a calming presleep routine
- Minimizing caffeine and sugar intake, especially in the evening
- Reducing screen time at least 1 hour before bed
- Ensuring a quiet, dark, and calm sleeping environment

These behavioral strategies can significantly reduce sleep latency and improve overall sleep quality. When behavioral strategies are insufficient, pharmacological interventions may be necessary. These may include [98–105]:

- Melatonin for circadian rhythm regulation
- Iron supplementation for RLS-related symptoms
- Clonidine or guanfacine for sedation and ADHD symptom control
- Modifying stimulant use to minimize sleep disruption
- Any pharmacological intervention must be supervised by a healthcare professional experienced in treating ADHD and sleep disorders.

Sleep disorders such as insomnia, restless leg syndrome, and delayed sleep phase disorder are frequently comorbid with ADHD and can significantly worsen its symptoms. A comprehensive treatment approach that includes behavioral strategies, sleep hygiene, and, when necessary, medical intervention is essential. Greater awareness and early intervention can break the cycle of poor sleep and impaired cognitive function, improving outcomes for individuals living with ADHD [86, 106, 107].

8.4 Multidisciplinary approach

It frequently co-occurs with a range of psychiatric, neurological, and physical health conditions, including anxiety, depression, learning disabilities, sleep disorders, and oppositional defiant disorder (ODD). These comorbidities complicate diagnosis and treatment and often require a coordinated, multidisciplinary approach to care. Collaboration among healthcare professionals, including pediatricians, psychiatrists, psychologists, neurologists, educators, occupational therapists, and sleep specialists, is essential for optimizing outcomes.

The symptoms of ADHD often overlap with or mask other conditions, making an accurate diagnosis complex. For example, mood disorders or anxiety may mimic inattentiveness or hyperactivity, while sleep disorders may exacerbate cognitive and behavioral symptoms of ADHD. These interconnected issues may go unrecognized or be misdiagnosed without a comprehensive evaluation.

8.5 Case coordination and communication

The multidisciplinary model is strongly characterized by collaboration in case management. All providers communicate regularly so that treatment goals are determined together and progress is tracked in a consistent manner. This kind of collaboration is particularly relevant with pediatric populations, since education requires collaboration between schools and families. Research has shown that collaborative care models lead to improved outcomes in children and adolescents with ADHD with comorbid conditions [108–110].

9. Treatment strategies

9.1 Comprehensive assessment

A comprehensive assessment is necessary to differentiate ADHD from other co-occurring psychological or developmental conditions, such as anxiety, depression, or learning disabilities. A correct diagnosis will allow interventions to be matched appropriately to fit the individual [111, 112].

9.2 Integrated treatment plans

A comprehensive treatment plan that includes both medication and behavioral strategies is generally viewed as the most effective way to manage ADHD symptoms. Evidence-based treatment options, both stimulant medications such as methylphenidate and amphetamines and non-stimulant medications such as atomoxetine, are available. These treatment options are even more effective when provided in a multimodal treatment plan that takes into account the individual needs of clients and includes other behavioral treatment alternatives such as cognitive behavioral therapy (CBT) and social skills training [52, 104, 111, 113–115].

9.3 Lifestyle modifications

Lifestyle factors play a critical role in managing ADHD symptoms. Regular physical activity, a balanced diet rich in omega-3 fatty acids, and mindfulness practices have been associated with improvements in attention, executive functioning, and emotional regulation [110, 116, 117].

9.4 Family and community support

Family involvement is vital in ADHD management. Psychoeducation programs, parent training interventions, and support groups can empower caregivers, reduce stress, and improve outcomes for children and adults with ADHD. Community-based services also provide essential resources and advocacy for ongoing support [118–120].

10. Conclusion

ADHD is rarely an isolated diagnosis; instead, it exists within a complex matrix of co-occurring conditions that demand a nuanced, multidisciplinary approach. The intersection of medical, psychological, educational, and social perspectives provides a robust foundation for comprehensive intervention. By fostering interdisciplinary collaboration, embracing personalized treatment strategies, and addressing the broader psychosocial context of ADHD, we can optimize outcomes and enhance the quality of life for individuals navigating the challenges of ADHD and its comorbidities. This chapter will further delve into the intricacies of ADHD's co-occurring conditions, examine best practices in diagnosis and intervention, and highlight the transformative potential of a multidisciplinary care model in advancing holistic well-being. Managing ADHD, particularly when accompanied by co-occurring conditions, requires more than a single-discipline approach. A coordinated, multidisciplinary team can provide the comprehensive care necessary for accurate diagnosis, effective treatment, and long-term success. As ADHD continues to be better understood, expanding access to collaborative models of care will be critical to improving outcomes for both children and adults.

Acknowledgements

This chapter would not have been possible without the support and encouragement of many individuals. I would first like to express my sincere gratitude to JB, whose guidance, feedback, and unwavering support helped shape the direction of this work.

Conflicts of interest

There are no conflicts of interest.

Abbreviations

ODD	oppositional defiant disorder
CBT	cognitive behavioral therapy
DSPD	delayed sleep phase disorder
RLS	restless leg syndrome
ASD	autism spectrum disorder
CD	conduct disorder

DOI: http://dx.doi.org/10.5772/intechopen.1011823

Author details

Jamuna Das and Jitendriya Biswal*
Department of Psychiatry, IMS and SUM Hospital (SOA Deemed to be University), Bhubaneswar, Odisha, India

*Address all correspondence to: drjbiswal@gmail.com

References

[1] Gnanavel S, Sharma P, Kaushal P, Hussain S. Attention deficit hyperactivity disorder and comorbidity: A review of literature. World Journal of Clinical Cases [Internet]. 2019;7(17):2420. Available from: https://pmc.ncbi.nlm.nih.gov/articles/PMC6745333/ [Accessed: March 17, 2025]

[2] Perrin JM, Stein MT, Amler RW, Blondis TA, Feldman HM, Meyer BP, et al. Clinical practice guideline: Treatment of the school-aged child with attention-deficit/hyperactivity disorder. Pediatrics. 2001;**108**(4):1033-1044

[3] van der Meer D, Hoekstra PJ, van Rooij D, Winkler AM, van Ewijk H, Heslenfeld DJ, et al. Anxiety modulates the relation between attention-deficit/hyperactivity disorder severity and working memory-related brain activity. The World Journal of Biological Psychiatry [Internet]. 2017;**19**(6):450. Available from: https://pmc.ncbi.nlm.nih.gov/articles/PMC5581282/ [Accessed: March 17, 2025]

[4] Hartman CA, Larsson H, Vos M, Bellato A, Libutzki B, Solberg BS, et al. Anxiety, mood, and substance use disorders in adult men and women with and without attention-deficit/hyperactivity disorder: A substantive and methodological overview. Neuroscience and Biobehavioral Reviews. 2023;**151**:105209

[5] Saccaro LF, Schilliger Z, Perroud N, Piguet C. Inflammation, anxiety, and stress in attention-deficit/hyperactivity disorder. Biomedicines [Internet]. 2021;**9**(10):1313. Available from: https://pmc.ncbi.nlm.nih.gov/articles/PMC8533349/ [Accessed: March 17, 2025]

[6] Morgenroth E, Saviola F, Gilleen J, Allen B, Lührs MW, Eysenck M, et al. Using connectivity-based real-time fMRI neurofeedback to modulate attentional and resting state networks in people with high trait anxiety. NeuroImage: Clinical. 1 Jan 2020;**25**. DOI: 10.1016/j.nicl.2020.102191 Epub ahead of print

[7] Meinzer MC, Chronis-Tuscano A. ADHD and the development of depression: Commentary on the prevalence, proposed mechanisms, and promising interventions. Current Developmental Disorders Reports [Internet]. 2017;**4**(1):1. Available from: https://pmc.ncbi.nlm.nih.gov/articles/PMC7717502/ [Accessed: March 17, 2025]

[8] Kita Y, Inoue Y. The direct/indirect association of ADHD/ODD symptoms with self-esteem, self-perception, and depression in early adolescents. Frontiers in Psychiatry [Internet]. 2017;**8**(JUL):137. Available from: https://pmc.ncbi.nlm.nih.gov/articles/PMC5534463/ [Accessed: March 17, 2025]

[9] Leitner Y. The co-occurrence of autism and attention deficit hyperactivity disorder in children - what do we know?. Frontiers in Human Neuroscience 29 Apr 2014;**8**:268. DOI: 10.3389/fnhum.2014.00268

[10] Davis NO, Kollins SH. Treatment for co-occurring attention deficit/hyperactivity disorder and autism spectrum disorder. Neurotherapeutics [Internet]. 2012;**9**(3):518-530. Available from: https://pubmed.ncbi.nlm.nih.gov/22678458/ [Accessed: March 17, 2025]

[11] Barry TD, Sturner R, Seymour K, Howard B, McGoron L, Bergmann P, et al. School-based screening to identify children at risk for attention-deficit/hyperactivity disorder: Barriers and

implications. Children's Health Care. 2016;**45**(3):241-265

[12] Chawla G, Juyal R, Shikha D, Semwal J, Tripathi S, Bhattacharya S. Attention deficit hyperactivity disorder and associated learning difficulties among primary school children in district Dehradun, Uttarakhand, India. Journal of Education and Health Promotion [Internet]. 2022;**11**(1):98. Available from: https://pmc.ncbi.nlm.nih.gov/articles/PMC9093659/ [Accessed: March 17, 2025]

[13] Steiner H, Remsing L, Work Group on Quality Issues. Practice parameter for the assessment and treatment of children and adolescents with oppositional defiant disorder. Journal of the American Academy of Child & Adolescent Psychiatry [Internet]. 2007;**46**(1):126-141. Available from: https://pubmed.ncbi.nlm.nih.gov/17195736/ [Accessed: March 17, 2025]

[14] Ahmad SI, Hinshaw SP. Attention-deficit/hyperactivity disorder, trait impulsivity, and externalizing behavior in a longitudinal sample. Journal of Abnormal Child Psychology [Internet]. 2017;**45**(6):1077. Available from: https://pmc.ncbi.nlm.nih.gov/articles/PMC5429206/ [Accessed: March 17, 2025]

[15] Shaw P, Stringaris A, Nigg J, Leibenluft E. Emotion dysregulation in attention deficit hyperactivity disorder. The American Journal of Psychiatry. 2014;**171**(3):276-293. DOI: 10.1176/appi.ajp.2013.13070966

[16] Zulauf CA, Sprich SE, Safren SA, Wilens TE. The complicated relationship between attention deficit/hyperactivity disorder and substance use disorders. Current Psychiatry Reports [Internet]. 2014;**16**(3):436. Available from: https://pmc.ncbi.nlm.nih.gov/articles/PMC4414493/ [Accessed: March 17, 2025]

[17] Molina BSG, Pelham WE. Attention-deficit/hyperactivity disorder and risk of substance use disorder: developmental considerations, potential pathways, and opportunities for research. Annual Review of Clinical Psychology. 2014;**10**:607-639. DOI: 10.1146/annurev-clinpsy-032813-153722

[18] Wilens TE, Spencer TJ. Understanding attention-deficit/hyperactivity disorder from childhood to adulthood. Postgraduate Medicine. 2010;**122**(5):97-109

[19] Havewala M, Lorenzo NE, Seddio K, Oddo LE, Novick DR, Fox NA, et al. Understanding Co-occurring ADHD and anxiety symptoms within a developmental framework: Risk and protective factors of early temperament and peer relations. Research on Child and Adolescent Psychopathology. 2022;**50**(7):853-866

[20] D'Agati E, Curatolo P, Mazzone L. Comorbidity between ADHD and anxiety disorders across the lifespan. International Journal of Psychiatry in Clinical Practice [Internet]. 2019;**23**(4):238-244. Available from: https://pubmed.ncbi.nlm.nih.gov/31232613/ [Accessed: March 19, 2025]

[21] Musser ED, Raiker JS. Attention-deficit/hyperactivity disorder: An integrated developmental psychopathology and research domain criteria (RDoC) approach. Comprehensive Psychiatry. 2019;**90**:65-72

[22] Wong RSY. Psychopathology of attention deficit/hyperactivity disorder: From an inflammatory perspective. The Egyptian Journal of Neurology, Psychiatry and Neurosurgery. 2022;**58**:123. DOI: 10.1186/s41983-022-00561-y

[23] Drechsler R, Brem S, Brandeis D, Grünblatt E, Berger G, Walitza S. ADHD: Current concepts and treatments in children and adolescents. Neuropediatrics [Internet]. 2020;**51**(5):315. Available from: https://pmc.ncbi.nlm.nih.gov/articles/PMC7508636/ [Accessed: March 19, 2025]

[24] Das J, Biswal J, Mohanty R. Exploring Emotional Regulation, Depression, Impulsivity, and Anxiety Connected to Attention Deficit Hyperactivity Disorder With Substance Use. Al-Rafidain Journal of Medical Sciences. Apr 2025;**8**(2):22-29. DOI: 10.54133/ajms.v8i2.1737. ISSN 2789-3219

[25] Schmidt S, Petermann F. Developmental psychopathology: Attention deficit hyperactivity disorder (ADHD). BMC Psychiatry [Internet]. 2009;**9**:58. Available from: https://pmc.ncbi.nlm.nih.gov/articles/PMC2751746/ [Accessed: March 19, 2025]

[26] Steinberg EA, Drabick DAG, Steinberg EA, Drabick DAG. A developmental psychopathology perspective on ADHD and comorbid conditions: The role of emotion regulation. Child Psychiatry & Human Development [Internet]. 2015;**46**(6):951-966. Available from: https://link.springer.com/article/10.1007/s10578-015-0534-2 [Accessed: March 19, 2025]

[27] Yadav SK, Bhat AA, Hashem S, Nisar S, Kamal M, Syed N, et al. Genetic variations influence brain changes in patients with attention-deficit hyperactivity disorder. Translational Psychiatry Psychiatry [Internet]. 2021;**11**(1):349. Available from: https://pmc.ncbi.nlm.nih.gov/articles/PMC8179928/ [Accessed: March 19, 2025]

[28] Martin EI, Ressler KJ, Binder E, Nemeroff CB. The neurobiology of anxiety disorders: Brain imaging, genetics, and Psychoneuroendocrinology. Psychiatric Clinics of North America [Internet]. 2009;**32**(3):549. Available from: https://pmc.ncbi.nlm.nih.gov/articles/PMC3684250/ [Accessed: March 19, 2025]

[29] Bush NR, Wakschlag LS, KZ LW, Hertz-Picciotto I, Nozadi SS, Pieper S, et al. Family environment, neurodevelopmental risk, and the environmental influences on child health outcomes (ECHO) initiative: Looking Back and moving forward. Frontiers in Psychiatry [Internet]. 2020;**11**:547. Available from: https://pmc.ncbi.nlm.nih.gov/articles/PMC7318113/ [Accessed: March 19, 2025]

[30] Froehlich TE, Anixt JS, Loe IM, Chirdkiatgumchai V, Kuan L, Gilman RC. Update on environmental risk factors for attention-deficit/hyperactivity disorder. Current Psychiatry Reports [Internet]. 2011;**13**(5):333. Available from: https://pmc.ncbi.nlm.nih.gov/articles/PMC3277258/ [Accessed: March 19, 2025]

[31] Lundervold AJ, Hinshaw SP, Sørensen L, Posserud MB. Co-occurring symptoms of attention deficit hyperactivity disorder (ADHD) in a population-based sample of adolescents screened for depression. BMC Psychiatry [Internet]. 2016;**16**(1):46. Available from: https://pmc.ncbi.nlm.nih.gov/articles/PMC4768418/ [Accessed: May 16, 2025]

[32] Riglin L, Leppert B, Dardani C, Thapar AK, Rice F, O'Donovan MC, et al. ADHD and depression: Investigating a causal explanation. Psychological Medicine [Internet]. 2020;**51**(11):1890. Available from: https://pmc.ncbi.nlm.nih.gov/articles/PMC8381237/ [Accessed: May 16, 2025]

[33] Chronis-Tuscano A, Molina BSG, Pelham WE, Applegate B, Dahlke A,

Overmyer M, et al. Very early predictors of adolescent depression and suicide attempts in children with attention-deficit/hyperactivity disorder. Archives of General Psychiatry. 2010;**67**(10):1044-1051

[34] Balbuena L, Bowen R, Baetz M, Marwaha S. Mood instability and irritability as core symptoms of major depression: An exploration using rasch analysis. Frontiers in Psychiatry. 26 Oct 2016;7. DOI: 10.3389/FPSYT.2016.00174 Epub ahead of print

[35] Gundel LK, Pedersen CB, Munk-Olsen T, Dalsgaard S. Longitudinal association between mental disorders in childhood and subsequent depression – A nationwide prospective cohort study. Journal of Affective Disorders. 2018;**227**:56-64

[36] Faraone SV, Larsson H. Genetics of attention deficit hyperactivity disorder. Molecular Psychiatry. 2019;**24**(4):562-575

[37] Bron TI, Bijlenga D, Verduijn J, Penninx BWJH, Beekman ATF, Kooij JJS. Prevalence of ADHD symptoms across clinical stages of major depressive disorder. Journal of Affective Disorders. 2016;**197**:29-35

[38] Cabral M, Demma I, et al. Attention-deficit/hyperactivity disorder: Diagnostic criteria, epidemiology, risk factors and evaluation in youth. Translational Pediatrics. 2020;**9**(Suppl 1):S104-S113. DOI: 10.21037/tp.2019.09.08

[39] Goodman DW, Thase ME. Recognizing ADHD in adults with comorbid mood disorders: Implications for identification and management. Postgraduate Medicine. 2009;**121**(5):31-41

[40] Eyre O, Langley K, Stringaris A, Leibenluft E, Collishaw S, Thapar A. Irritability in ADHD: Associations with depression liability. Journal of Affective Disorders. 2017;**215**:281-287

[41] Sadeghian Nadooshan MR, Shahrivar Z, Mahmoudi Gharaie J, Salehi L. ADHD in adults with major depressive or bipolar disorder: Does it affect clinical features, comorbidity, quality of life, and global functioning? BMC Psychiatry [Internet]. 2022;**22**(1):707. Available from: https://pmc.ncbi.nlm.nih.gov/articles/PMC9667673/ [Accessed: March 19, 2025]

[42] Kuś J, Saramowicz K, Czerniawska M, Wiese W, Siwecka N, Rozpędek-Kamińska W, et al. Molecular mechanisms underlying NMDARs dysfunction and their role in ADHD pathogenesis. International Journal of Molecular Sciences [Internet]. 2023;**24**(16):12983. Available from: https://www.mdpi.com/1422-0067/24/16/12983/htm [Accessed: March 20, 2025]

[43] Hurley AD, Levitas AS, Bertelli MO. Mood Disorder. In: Textbook of Psychiatry for Intellectual Disability and Autism Spectrum Disorder [Internet]. Treasure Island (FL): StatPearls Publishing; 2023. pp. 557-581. Available from: https://www.ncbi.nlm.nih.gov/books/NBK558911/ [Accessed: March 20, 2025]

[44] Salvi V, Ribuoli E, Servasi M, Orsolini L, Volpe U. ADHD and bipolar disorder in adulthood: Clinical and treatment implications. Medicina (B Aires) [Internet]. 2021;**57**(5):466. Available from: https://pmc.ncbi.nlm.nih.gov/articles/PMC8151516/ [Accessed: March 20, 2025]

[45] Hirsch O, Chavanon ML, Christiansen H. Emotional dysregulation subgroups in patients with adult

attention-deficit/hyperactivity disorder (ADHD): A cluster analytic approach. Scientific Reports. 1 Dec 2019;**9**(1). DOI: 10.1038/S41598-019-42018-Y Epub ahead of print

[46] Swann AC, Moeller FG, Steinberg JL, Schneider L, Barratt ES, Dougherty DM. Manic symptoms and impulsivity during bipolar depressive episodes. Bipolar Disorders [Internet]. 2007;**9**(3):206. Available from: https://pmc.ncbi.nlm.nih.gov/articles/PMC2723749/ [Accessed: March 20, 2025]

[47] Corbisiero S, Riecher-Rössler A, Buchli-Kammermann J, Stieglitz RD. Symptom overlap and screening for symptoms of attention-deficit/hyperactivity disorder and psychosis risk in help-seeking psychiatric patients. Frontiers in Psychiatry [Internet]. 2017;**8**(OCT):290604. Available from: www.frontiersin.org [Accessed: March 20, 2025]

[48] Lopez PL, Torrente FM, Ciapponi A, Lischinsky AG, Cetkovich-Bakmas M, Rojas JI, et al. Cognitive-behavioural interventions for attention deficit hyperactivity disorder (ADHD) in adults. Cochrane Database of Systematic Reviews [Internet]. 2018;**2018**(3):CD010840. Available from: https://pmc.ncbi.nlm.nih.gov/articles/PMC6494390/ [Accessed: April 22, 2025]

[49] Ryum T, Kazantzis N. Elucidating the process-based emphasis in cognitive behavioral therapy. Journal of Contextual Behavioral Science. 2024;**33**:100819

[50] Snowling MJ, Hulme C, Nation K. Defining and understanding dyslexia: Past, present and future. Oxford Review of Education [Internet]. 2020;**46**(4):501. Available from: https://pmc.ncbi.nlm.nih.gov/articles/PMC7455053/ [Accessed: April 22, 2025]

[51] Haberstroh S, Schulte-Körne G. The diagnosis and treatment of dyscalculia. Deutsches Ärzteblatt International [Internet]. 2019;**116**(7):107. Available from: https://pmc.ncbi.nlm.nih.gov/articles/PMC6440373/ [Accessed: April 22, 2025]

[52] Wehmeier PM, Schacht A, Barkley RA. Social and emotional impairment in children and adolescents with ADHD and the impact on quality of life. Journal of Adolescent Health [Internet]. 2010;**46**(3):209-217. Available from: https://www.sciencedirect.com/science/article/abs/pii/S1054139X09003784 [Accessed: May 8, 2025]

[53] McDonough EM, Flanagan DP, Sy M, Alfonso VC. Specific learning disorder. In: Handbook of DSM-5 Disorders in Children and Adolescents [Internet]. Cham: Springer; 2017. pp. 77-104. Available from: http://link.springer.com/10.1007/978-3-319-57196-6_4 [Accessed: May 8, 2025]

[54] Azeredo A, Moreira D, Barbosa F. ADHD, CD, and ODD: Systematic review of genetic and environmental risk factors. Research in Developmental Disabilities [Internet]. 2018;**82**:10-19. Available from: https://www.sciencedirect.com/science/article/abs/pii/S0891422217303177 [Accessed: May 9, 2025]

[55] Ghosh S, Sinha M. ADHD, ODD, and CD: Do they belong to a common psychopathological Spectrum? A case series. Case Reports in Psychiatry [Internet]. 2012;**2012**:520689. Available from: https://pmc.ncbi.nlm.nih.gov/articles/PMC3477532/ [Accessed: May 9, 2025]

[56] Burke JD, Butler EJ, Blanchard L. Oppositional defiant disorder. In: Encyclopedia of Mental Health, Third

Edition: Volume 1-3 [Internet]. Vol. 2. Treasure Island (FL): StatPearls Publishing; 2024. pp. V2-683-V2-691. Available from: https://www.ncbi.nlm.nih.gov/books/NBK557443/ [Accessed: May 9, 2025]

[57] Anney RJL et al. Conduct disorder and ADHD: Evaluation of conduct problems as a categorical and quantitative trait in the international multicentre ADHD genetics study. American journal of medical genetics. Part B, Neuropsychiatric genetics: The official publication of the International Society of Psychiatric Genetics. 2008;**147B**(8):1369-1378. DOI: 10.1002/ajmg.b.30871

[58] Matthys W, Vanderschuren LJMJ, Schutter DJLG. The neurobiology of oppositional defiant disorder and conduct disorder: Altered functioning in three mental domains. Development and Psychopathology. 2013;**25**(1):193-207

[59] Rowe R, Costello EJ, Angold A, Copeland WE, Maughan B. Developmental pathways in oppositional defiant disorder and conduct disorder. Journal of Abnormal Psychology [Internet]. 2010;**119**(4):726. Available from: https://pmc.ncbi.nlm.nih.gov/articles/PMC3057683/ [Accessed: May 9, 2025]

[60] Maughan B, Rowe R, Messer J, Goodman R, Meltzer H. Conduct disorder and oppositional defiant disorder in a national sample: Developmental epidemiology. Journal of Child Psychology and Psychiatry, and Allied Disciplines. 2004;**45**(3):609-621. DOI: 10.1111/j.1469-7610.2004.00250.x

[61] Helander M, Enebrink P, Hellner C, Ahlen J. Parent management training combined with group-CBT compared to parent management training only for oppositional defiant disorder symptoms: 2-year follow-up of a randomized controlled trial. Child Psychiatry & Human Development [Internet]. 2022;**54**(4):1112. Available from: https://pmc.ncbi.nlm.nih.gov/articles/PMC10271908/ [Accessed: May 9, 2025]

[62] Pfiffner LJ, Haack LM. Behavior Management for School Aged Children with ADHD. Child and Adolescent Psychiatric Clinics of North America [Internet]. 2014;**23**(4):731. Available from: https://pmc.ncbi.nlm.nih.gov/articles/PMC4167345/ [Accessed: May 9, 2025]

[63] Mechler K, Banaschewski T, Hohmann S, Häge A. Evidence-based pharmacological treatment options for ADHD in children and adolescents. Pharmacology & Therapeutics [Internet]. 2022;**230**:107940. Available from: https://www.sciencedirect.com/science/article/pii/S016372582100142X [Accessed: May 9, 2025]

[64] Hood BS, Elrod MG, DeWine DB. Treatment of childhood oppositional defiant disorder. Current Treatment Options in Pediatrics [Internet]. 2015;**1**(2):155-167. Available from: https://link.springer.com/article/10.1007/s40746-015-0015-7 [Accessed: May 9, 2025]

[65] Al Ghamdi K, Almusailhi J. Attention-deficit hyperactivity disorder and autism Spectrum disorder: Towards better diagnosis and management. Medical Archives [Internet]. 2024;**78**(2):159. Available from: https://pmc.ncbi.nlm.nih.gov/articles/PMC10983102/ [Accessed: May 9, 2025]

[66] Craig F, Lamanna AL, Margari F, Matera E, Simone M, Margari L. Overlap between autism Spectrum disorders and attention deficit hyperactivity disorder: Searching for distinctive/common clinical features. Autism Research

[Internet]. 2015;**8**(3):328. Available from: https://pmc.ncbi.nlm.nih.gov/articles/PMC4654237/ [Accessed: May 9, 2025]

[67] Tager-Flusberg H, Caronna E. Language disorders: Autism and other pervasive developmental disorders. Pediatric Clinics of North America. 2007;**54**(3):469-481

[68] Farmer M, Oliver A. Assessment of pragmatic difficulties and socio-semotional adjustment in practice. International Journal of Language & Communication Disorders. 2005;**40**(4):403-429

[69] Bishop DVM, Baird G. Parent and teacher report of pragmatic aspects of communication: Use of the children's communication checklist in a clinical setting. Developmental Medicine & Child Neurology [Internet]. 2001;**43**(12):809. Available from: https://pubmed.ncbi.nlm.nih.gov/11769267/ [Accessed: May 9, 2025]

[70] Ramtekkar UP. DSM-5 changes in attention deficit hyperactivity disorder and autism Spectrum disorder: Implications for comorbid sleep issues. Children [Internet]. 2017;**4**(8):62. Available from: https://pmc.ncbi.nlm.nih.gov/articles/PMC5575584/ [Accessed: May 9, 2025]

[71] Theodoratou M. Communication issues in co-occurring ADHD and autism spectrum disorders. Evaluative approaches and targeted interventions: Mini review. Advances in Psychiatry and Neurology [Internet]. 2024;**33**(3):188. Available from: https://pmc.ncbi.nlm.nih.gov/articles/PMC11635427/ [Accessed: May 9, 2025]

[72] Verma B, Dey M, Sehgal R. Exploring Prevalence of Sensory Patterns Among Children With Developmental Disabilities: A Cross-Sectional Study. International Journal of Contemporary Pediatrics. Feb 2025;**12**(3):471-478. DOI: 10.18203/2349-3291.ijcp20250413

[73] Alenezi S, Alkhiri A, Hassanin W, AlHarbi A, Al Assaf M, Alzunaydi N, et al. Findings of a multidisciplinary assessment of children referred for possible neurodevelopmental disorders: Insights from a retrospective chart review study. Behavioral Sciences [Internet]. 2022;**12**(12):509. Available from: https://www.mdpi.com/2076-328X/12/12/509/htm [Accessed: May 9, 2025]

[74] Young S, Hollingdale J, Absoud M, Bolton P, Branney P, Colley W, et al. Guidance for identification and treatment of individuals with attention deficit/hyperactivity disorder and autism spectrum disorder based upon expert consensus. BMC Medicine [Internet]. 2020;**18**(1):146. Available from: https://pmc.ncbi.nlm.nih.gov/articles/PMC7247165/ [Accessed: May 9, 2025]

[75] Samal B, Senjam G, Ravan J, Ningombam H, Das R, Das S. Prevalence of adult ADHD in patients with substance use disorder in north East India. ndian Journal of Psychiatry [Internet]. 2022;**31**(2):214. Available from: https://pubmed.ncbi.nlm.nih.gov/36419685/ [Accessed: July 26, 2024]

[76] Ohlmeier MD, Goseberg E, Roy M, Dillo W, Kordon A, Prox-Vagedes V. Alcohol and drug dependence in adults with attention-deficit/hyperactivity disorder: Data from Germany. The European Journal of Psychiatry [Internet]. 2011;**25**(3):150-163. Available from: https://scielo.isciii.es/scielo.php?script=sci_arttext&pid=S0213-61632011000300005&lng=es&nrm=iso&tlng=en [Accessed: May 9, 2025]

[77] Young S, Abbasian C, Al-Attar Z, Branney P, Colley B, Cortese S,

et al. Identification and treatment of individuals with attention-deficit/hyperactivity disorder and substance use disorder: An expert consensus statement. World Journal of Psychiatry. 19 Mar 2023;**13**(3):84-112. DOI: 10.5498/wjp.v13.i3.84

[78] Zulauf CA, Sprich SE, Safren SA, Wilens TE. The complicated relationship between attention deficit/hyperactivity disorder and substance use disorders topical collection on child and adolescent disorders. Current Psychiatry Reports. 2014;**16**(3):436. DOI: 10.1007/s11920-013-0436-6

[79] Spera V, Pallucchini A, Maiello M, Carli M, Maremmani AGI, Perugi G, et al. Substance use disorder in adult-attention deficit hyperactive disorder patients: patterns of use and related clinical features. International Journal of Environmental Research and Public Health. 17 May. 2020;**17**(10):3509 DOI: 10.3390/ijerph17103509

[80] Shier AC, Reichenbacher T, Ghuman HS, Ghuman JK. Pharmacological treatment of attention deficit hyperactivity disorder in children and adolescents: Clinical strategies. Journal of Central Nervous System Disease [Internet]. 2012;**5**:1. Available from: https://pmc.ncbi.nlm.nih.gov/articles/PMC3616598/ [Accessed: May 9, 2025]

[81] Volkow ND, Swanson JM. Does childhood treatment of ADHD with stimulant medication affect substance abuse in adulthood? American Journal of Psychiatry [Internet]. 2008;**165**(5):553. Available from: https://pmc.ncbi.nlm.nih.gov/articles/PMC2667111/ [Accessed: May 9, 2025]

[82] Young S, Yoon R, Jain U, Shapiro C. CLINICAL REVIEW sleep in attention-deficit/hyperactivity disorder in children and adults: Past, present, and future. Sleep Medicine Reviews. 2012;**16**(4):371-388

[83] Sung V, Hiscock H, Sciberras E, Efron D. Sleep problems in children with attention-deficit/hyperactivity disorder: Prevalence and the effect on the child and family. Archives of Pediatrics & Adolescent Medicine. 2008;**162**(4):336-342

[84] Um YH, Hong SC, Jeong JH. Sleep problems as predictors in attention-deficit hyperactivity disorder: Causal mechanisms, consequences and treatment. Clinical Psychopharmacology and Neuroscience [Internet]. 2017;**15**(1):9. Available from: https://pmc.ncbi.nlm.nih.gov/articles/PMC5290714/ [Accessed: May 9, 2025]

[85] Stein MA, Weiss M, Hlavaty L. ADHD treatments, sleep, and sleep problems: Complex associations. Neurotherapeutics [Internet]. 2012;**9**(3):509. Available from: https://pmc.ncbi.nlm.nih.gov/articles/PMC3441938/ [Accessed: May 9, 2025]

[86] Wajszilber D, Santiseban JA, Gruber R. Sleep disorders in patients with ADHD: Impact and management challenges. Nature and Science of Sleep. 2018;**10**:453-480

[87] Bjorvatn B, Brevik EJ, Lundervold AJ, Halmøy A, Posserud MB, Instanes JT, et al. Adults with attention deficit hyperactivity disorder report high symptom levels of troubled sleep, restless legs, and cataplexy. Frontiers in Psychology. 20 Sep 2017;**8**:1621. DOI: 10.3389/fpsyg.2017.01621

[88] Murawski B, Wade L, Plotnikoff RC, Lubans DR, Duncan MJ. A systematic review and meta-analysis of cognitive and behavioral interventions to improve sleep health in adults without sleep disorders. Sleep Medicine Review

[Internet]. 2018;**40**:160-169. Available from: https://www.sciencedirect.com/science/article/pii/S1087079217301661 [Accessed: May 9, 2025]

[89] Jernelöv S, Larsson Y, Llenas M, Nasri B, Kaldo V. Effects and clinical feasibility of a behavioral treatment for sleep problems in adult attention deficit hyperactivity disorder (ADHD): A pragmatic within-group pilot evaluation. BMC Psychiatry [Internet]. 2019;**19**(1):226. Available from: https://bmcpsychiatry.biomedcentral.com/articles/10.1186/s12888-019-2216-2 [Accessed: May 9, 2025]

[90] Migueis DP, Lopes MC, Casella E, Soares P V, Soster L, Spruyt K. Attention deficit hyperactivity disorder and restless leg syndrome across the lifespan: A systematic review and meta-analysis. Sleep Medicine Reviews. 2023;**69**:101770. DOI: 10.1016/J.SMRV.2023.101770

[91] Konofal E, Cortese S, Marchand M, Mouren MC, Arnulf I, Lecendreux M. Impact of restless legs syndrome and iron deficiency on attention-deficit/hyperactivity disorder in children. Sleep Medivine [Internet]. 2007;**8**(7-8):711-715. Available from: https://pubmed.ncbi.nlm.nih.gov/17644481/ [Accessed: May 13, 2025]

[92] Futenma K, Takaesu Y, Komada Y, Shimura A, Okajima I, Matsui K, et al. Delayed sleep–wake phase disorder and its related sleep behaviors in the young generation. Frontiers in Psychiatry [Internet]. 2023;**14**:1174719. Available from: https://pmc.ncbi.nlm.nih.gov/articles/PMC10235460/ [Accessed: May 13, 2025]

[93] Van Veen MM, Kooij JJS, Boonstra AM, Gordijn MCM, Van Someren EJW. Delayed circadian rhythm in adults with attention-deficit/hyperactivity disorder and chronic sleep-onset insomnia. Biological Psychiatry [Internet]. 2010;**67**(11):1091-1096. Available from: https://pubmed.ncbi.nlm.nih.gov/20163790/ [Accessed: May 13, 2025]

[94] Ophoff D, Slaats MA, Boudewyns A, Glazemakers I, Van Hoorenbeeck K, Verhulst SL. Sleep disorders during childhood: A practical review. European Journal of Pediatrics. 2018;**177**(5):641-648

[95] Yin H, Yang D, Yang L, Wu G. Relationship between sleep disorders and attention-deficit-hyperactivity disorder in children. Frontiers in Pediatrics. 22 Jul 2022;**10**:919572. DOI: 10.3389/fped.2022.919572

[96] French B, Quain E, Kilgariff J, Lockwood J, Daley D. The impact of sleep difficulties in children with attention deficit hyperactivity disorder on the family: A thematic analysis. Journal of Clinical Sleep Medicine [Internet]. 2023;**19**(10):1735. Available from: https://pmc.ncbi.nlm.nih.gov/articles/PMC10545997/ [Accessed: May 13, 2025]

[97] Posner D, Gehrman PR. Sleep Hygiene. Behavioral Treatments for Sleep Disorders; 2011. pp. 31-43. DOI: 10.1016/B978-0-12-381522-4.00003-1

[98] Stein MA et al. ADHD treatments, sleep, and sleep problems: complex associations. Neurotherapeutics: the Journal of the American Society for Experimental NeuroTherapeutics. 2012;**9**(3):509-517. DOI: 10.1007/s13311-012-0130-0

[99] Rigney G, Ali NS, Corkum PV, Brown CA, Constantin E, Godbout R, et al. A systematic review to explore the feasibility of a behavioural sleep intervention for insomnia in children with neurodevelopmental disorders: A transdiagnostic approach. Sleep Medicine Reviews. 2018;**41**:244-254

[100] O'Regan D, Anderson KN. Restless legs syndrome and periodic limb movements of sleep. British Journal of Hospital Medicine (London, England). 2020;**81**(1):1-8

[101] Mammarella V et al. Pharmacological management for insomnia in children and adolescents with autism and attention deficit and hyperactivity disorder. Expert Opinion on Pharmacotherapy. 2025;**26**(9):1079-1098. DOI: 10.1080/14656566.2025.2508277

[102] Devnani P. Sleep Disorders. International Journal of Head and Neck Surgery [Internet]. 2019;**10**(1):4-8. Available from: https://www.ijhns.com/doi/10.5005/jp-journals-10001-1362 [Accessed: May 13, 2025]

[103] Dimakos J, Giorgio LM, Gruber R. Sleep and Attention-Deficit/Hyperactivity Disorder. In: Gupta R, Neubauer DN, Pandi-Perumal SR, editors. Sleep and Neuropsychiatric Disorders. Singapore: Springer; 2022. pp. 523-54 DOI: 10.1007/978-981-16-0123-1_25

[104] Voysey ZJ, Barker RA, Lazar AS. The treatment of sleep dysfunction in neurodegenerative disorders. Neurotherapeutics. 2021;**18**(1):202-216

[105] Tamir S, Dye TJ, Witt RM. Sleep and circadian disturbances in children with neurodevelopmental disorders. Seminars in Pediatric Neurology. 2023;**48**:101090. DOI: 10.1016/j.spen.2023.101090

[106] Gau SSF, Kessler RC, Tseng WL, Wu YY, Chiu YN, Bin YC, et al. Association between sleep problems and symptoms of attention-deficit/hyperactivity disorder in young adults. Sleep. 2007;**30**(2):195-201

[107] Corkum P, Tannock R, Moldofsky H. Sleep disturbances in children with attention-deficit/hyperactivity disorder. Journal of the American Academy of Child and Adolescent Psychiatry. 1998;**37**(6):637-646

[108] Couturier Y, Lanoue S, Karam M, Guillette M, Hudon C. Social workers coordination in primary healthcare for patients with complex needs: A scoping review. International Journal of Care Coordination. 2023;**26**(1):5-25

[109] Talbott E, De Los RA, Power TJ, Michel JJ, Racz SJ. A team-based collaborative care model for youth with attention-deficit hyperactivity disorder in education and health care settings. Journal of Emotional and Behavioral Disorders. 2021;**29**(1):24-33

[110] Visser SN, Danielson ML, Bitsko RH, Holbrook JR, Kogan MD, Ghandour RM, et al. Trends in the parent-report of health care provider-diagnosed and medicated attention-deficit/hyperactivity disorder: United States, 2003-2011. Journal of the American Academy of Child and Adolescent Psychiatry. 2014;**53**(1):34-46.e2. DOI: 10.1016/j.jaac.2013.09.001

[111] Salari N, Ghasemi H, Abdoli N, Rahmani A, Shiri MH, Hashemian AH, et al. The global prevalence of ADHD in children and adolescents: A systematic review and meta-analysis. Ital. The Journal of Pediatrics. 20 Apr 2023;**49**(1):48. DOI: 10.1186/s13052-023-01456-1

[112] Wilens, Timothy E et al. Attention-deficit/hyperactivity disorder and transitional aged youth. Current Psychiatry Reports. 17 Sep 2018;**20**(11):100. DOI: 10.1007/s11920-018-0968-x

[113] Brown KA, Samuel S, Patel DR. Pharmacologic management of attention

deficit hyperactivity disorder in children and adolescents: A review for practitioners. Translational Pediatrics [Internet]. 2018;7(1):36. Available from: https://pmc.ncbi.nlm.nih.gov/articles/PMC5803014/ [Accessed: May 13, 2025]

[114] Young S, Absoud M, Al-Attar Z, Ani C, Colley W, Cortese S, et al. The ADHD assessment quality assurance standard for children and teenagers (CAAQAS). Neuropsychiatric Disease and Treatment [Internet]. 2024;**20**:2603-2628. Available from: https://www.dovepress.com/the-adhd-assessment-quality-assurance-standard-for-children-and-teenag-peer-reviewed-fulltext-article-NDT [Accessed: May 13, 2025]

[115] Wolraich M, Brown L, Brown RT, DuPaul G, Earls M, Feldman HM, et al. ADHD: Clinical practice guideline for the diagnosis, evaluation, and treatment of attention-deficit/hyperactivity disorder in children and adolescents. Pediatrics. 2011;**128**(5):1007-1022

[116] Wolraich ML, Hagan JF, Allan C, Chan E, Davison D, Earls M, et al. Clinical practice guideline for the diagnosis, evaluation, and treatment of attention-deficit/hyperactivity disorder in children and adolescents. Pediatrics. 2019;**144**(4):e20192528. DOI: 10.1542/peds. 2019-2528

[117] Shrestha M, Lautenschleger J, Soares N. Non-pharmacologic management of attention-deficit/hyperactivity disorder in children and adolescents: A review. Translational Pediatrics [Internet]. 2020;**9**(Suppl 1):S114. Available from: https://pmc.ncbi.nlm.nih.gov/articles/PMC7082245/ [Accessed: May 13, 2025]

[118] Abikoff H, Hechtman L, Klein RG, Gallagher R, Fleiss K, Etcovitch J, et al. Social functioning in children with ADHD treated with long-term methylphenidate and multimodal psychosocial treatment. Journal of the American Academy of Child and Adolescent Psychiatry. 2004;**43**(7):820-829

[119] Zwi M, Jones H, Thorgaard C, York A, Dennis JA. Parent training interventions for attention deficit hyperactivity disorder (ADHD) in children aged 5 to 18 years. Cochrane Database of Systematic Reviews [Internet]. 2011;**2011**(12):CD003018. Available from: https://pmc.ncbi.nlm.nih.gov/articles/PMC6544776/ [Accessed: May 13, 2025]

[120] Mikami AY, Jack A, Emeh CC, Stephens HF. Parental influence on children with attention-deficit/hyperactivity disorder: I. Relationships between parent behaviors and child peer status. Journal of Abnormal Child Psychology. 2010;**38**(6):721-736

Chapter 6

Updates on ADHD in Children and Adolescents: Approach to Diagnosis and Management

Madeeha Kamal and Khoulod Mohamed

Abstract

Attention-deficit/hyperactivity disorder (ADHD) is a prevalent neurodevelopmental condition affecting individuals across the lifespan. It has considerable implications for academic, social, and occupational functioning. The prevalence varies across genders, populations, and different age groups. Accurate diagnosis involves comprehensive clinical assessment and is mainly based on the updated criteria of the Diagnostic and Statistical Manual of Mental Disorders (DSM)-5th edition (DSM-5). ADHD can co-occur with other conditions, such as autism, learning disabilities, and mood disorders, which can complicate the clinical presentation and management process. Management of ADHD should be well-planned, with shared decision-making between healthcare teams, patients, families, and school personnel to address individual needs and encourage compliance. It combines pharmacological therapies, including stimulant and non-stimulant medications, along with behavioral therapies. Multidisciplinary approaches are critical for improving outcomes and minimizing the impact of symptoms. Without proper early diagnosis and management, individuals with ADHD are at high risk for long-term complications on multiple levels at different ages, including academic underachievement, poor social functioning, and comorbidities, resulting in overall dissatisfaction. As our understanding of ADHD evolves, further research is vital to refine diagnostic and treatment approaches and improve the quality of life for affected individuals.

Keywords: attention deficit hyperactivity disorder (ADHD), children, adolescents, diagnosis, comorbidities, management, impacts

1. Introduction

1.1 Overview

Attention-deficit/hyperactivity disorder (ADHD) is a common neurodevelopmental condition that results in lifelong complications and impairs quality of life on multiple levels. Without timely diagnosis and management, it can lead to significant limitations of social, academic, and professional performances with irreversible impacts, and can increase the chance of comorbid conditions that further compromise well-being and complicate management. It is characterized by different forms of developmentally inappropriate levels of inattention, hyperactivity and/or impulsivity that influence the ability to reach sustained concentration, organize tasks and responsibilities, or regulate behavior and responses as per social norms and expectations.

ADHD is a dynamic disorder that calls for constant updates in our knowledge on diagnosis and management to prevent missed cases or late diagnoses that put affected individuals at risk of unchangeable life conditions. ADHD should not be regarded as a childhood disorder, as it can persist into adulthood and continue to exert limitations on both personal and professional levels. In addition, it can affect apparently healthy individuals who rarely seek medical care for acute conditions. Accordingly, healthcare providers should remain vigilant and attentive to features of the disorder in order to identify cases as early as possible. Moreover, healthcare providers should raise the population's awareness of the condition and its features to increase the chance of case identification at any setting and consequent direction to appropriate management.

1.2 Aim

In this chapter, we are going to explore the burden of ADHD in terms of the prevalence and distribution and to examine its core symptoms and diagnostic criteria. We will also discuss the challenges associated with ADHD in different life stages, review that latest management approaches, ranging from behavioral therapies to medications, and highlight the potential comorbidities.

2. Epidemiology

2.1 Prevalence

ADHD is commonly diagnosed in children and adolescents. It is regarded as the most common behavioral condition [1]. The prevalence is rising with increasing awareness of diagnostic criteria among healthcare providers and the society, including caregivers, and with the availability of effective management that yields promising life-changing results [2]. According to a meta-analysis conducted by Ayano and his colleagues in 2023, the pooled international prevalence of ADHD is around 8%, with a range of 3.4–14% based on epidemiology studies from different developed and developing countries across the globe. Remarkably, there is a relatively higher prevalence of ADHD among American, Indian, and Middle Eastern populations by 1.5–2.5 times in comparison with other populations like African, Chinese, or European populations. In Qatar, our country of practice, a study in 2014 showed that as many as 19% of Qatari children between the ages of 6 and 12 in government schools have moderate to high levels of ADHD [3–5].

2.2 Gender distribution

Boys are more commonly diagnosed with ADHD compared to girls. It has been repeatedly highlighted in literature that the diagnostic and referral rates for ADHD show a clear gender difference, with the ratio of boys to girls diagnosed or referred with ADHD ranging from 2:1 to 10:1 [6]. This is largely explained by the nature of presenting symptoms in both genders. Boys are more likely to present with disruptive, predominantly hyperactive, and/or impulsive symptoms along with associated behavioral disorders. In contrast, girls are more likely to present with inattentiveness and are more likely to internalize symptoms due to potential comorbidities, such as anxiety or depression. In addition, some studies pointed to the theory of "female protective effect" to explain the gender difference. This theory indicates that females need a higher load of genetic and environmental factors to manifest the same degree of impairment demonstrated by males [7, 8].

2.3 Subtypes and persistence rates

In terms of subtypes of ADHD, the review of Ayano et al. showed that the inattentive type is the commonest type inattentive type with a prevalence of 3%, followed by the hyperactive type and the combined type with a prevalence of 2.95 and 2.44%, respectively [3]. This is potentially due to the consistent nature of inattentive symptoms over time. However, hyperactive and impulsive symptoms are more likely to improve with age [9]. The prevalence of ADHD tends to decrease with age. It has been shown that the prevalence of ADHD in adolescence is about half of that in childhood. Similarly, the estimates continue to decrease in adulthood. It has been reported that estimated prevalence of ADHD during childhood decreases from 5 to 7 to 3–5% in adulthood. Nevertheless, these data should be interpreted with caution since the topic of ADHD has less research attention in the adult age group, which may underestimate the real burden of the disease in adults [10].

Sibley and her colleagues reviewed the rates of ADHD persistence into adulthood as per several longitudinal studies and reported a largely heterogeneous rate of 5–75%. This heterogeneity could be brought about by variations in study samples, definitions of persistence, sources, and methods used, and thresholds for reporting symptoms [11]. Caye et al. discussed that females can have a higher persistence rate into adulthood compared to males, along with higher chances of negative outcomes. Interestingly, they pointed that clinically significant ADHD symptoms and resulting impairments can start after childhood, which alters the perception of ADHD as a neurodevelopmental condition with an exclusive onset during childhood [12].

3. Diagnosis

3.1 Diagnostic criteria

The diagnostic criteria of ADHD, according to the Diagnostic and Statistical Manual of Mental Disorders (DSM)-5th edition (DSM-5), were last revised in 2013 to increase the diagnostic reliability. According to the manual, ADHD can be diagnosed in the presence of the following: six or more symptoms of inattention and/or hyperactivity-impulsivity for children up to 16 years of age or five or more symptoms of inattention and/or hyperactivity/impulsivity for adolescents aged 17 years and older, or adults. Symptoms should be present for at least 6 months and should be inappropriate for the individual's developmental level.

In addition, the following features should be applicable: Several symptoms should be present before the age of 12 years, several symptoms are present in two or more settings (such as at home, school or work; with friends or relatives; in other activities), symptoms clearly interfere with or reduce the quality of social, academic, or occupational functioning, symptoms are not better explained by another mental disorder (such as a mood disorder, anxiety disorder, dissociative disorder, or a personality disorder), and symptoms do not happen only during the course of schizophrenia or another psychotic disorder. ADHD is classified in the DSM-5 into predominantly inattentive, predominantly impulsive or hyperactive or combined presentation [13, 14].

A patient with inattentive symptoms often exhibits the following behaviors: Fails to give close attention to details or makes careless mistakes in schoolwork, at work, or with other activities, has trouble holding attention on tasks or play activities, does not seem to listen when spoken to directly, does not follow through on instructions and fails to finish schoolwork, chores, or duties in the workplace (e.g., loses focus, side-tracked), has trouble organizing tasks and activities, avoids, dislikes, or is reluctant to do tasks that require mental effort over a long period of time (such as schoolwork or homework), loses things necessary for tasks and activities (e.g., school materials, pencils, books, tools, wallets, keys, paperwork, eyeglasses, mobile telephones), is easily distracted, and/or is forgetful in daily activities [13, 15].

A patient with hyperactive/impulsive symptoms often exhibits the following behaviors: Fidgets with or taps hands or feet, or squirms in seat, leaves seat in situations when remaining seated is expected, feels restless or runs about or climbs in situations where it is not appropriate, is unable to play or take part in leisure activities quietly, is "on the go" acting as if "driven by a motor," talks excessively, blurts out an answer before a question has been completed, has trouble waiting their turn, and/or interrupts or intrudes on others (e.g., butts into conversations or games) [13].

3.2 Evaluation process

The evaluation and diagnosis of ADHD should be based on detailed history taking, since there are no investigations available to support diagnosis. Neuropsychological tests are not as sensitive as history taking in formulating the diagnosis. History should be gathered using different rating scales and should be elicited from multiple informants, like parents and teachers, to assess the universality of symptoms in different settings. In addition, history taking should aim at gathering information about potential risk factors of ADHD. It has a multifactorial etiology that includes both genetic and environmental components. ADHD is considered one of the most heritable conditions in terms of psychiatric disorders, and siblings of affected individuals have a higher risk of developing the condition compared to the general population. Besides genetics, some environmental factors have been shown to increase the risk of ADHD, such as viral infections, extremely low birth weight, smoking or alcoholism during pregnancy, and malnutrition [16].

There are different scales available to gather information in the process of ADHD evaluation. The Vanderbilt scale is often used with children and adolescents as it has both parent and teacher components. Other rating scales include Conner's scale and Brown attention-deficit disorder, which can be used for different age groups, including adults [17, 18]. The role of physical examination and investigations in diagnosing ADHD is limited to the exclusion of medical conditions that could mimic ADHD symptoms, such as thyroid disorders, anemia, seizure disorders, or sensory processing disorders. In addition, some medical conditions may influence treatment choices of ADHD, like hypertension that disfavors the use of stimulant medications [16, 19, 20].

3.3 Etiology

There has been no consensus so far on the neurobiological basis of ADHD. Studies highlighted the presence of a correlation between ADHD and neuroimaging findings of white matter abnormalities in cortico-striatal pathways and the prefrontal cortex. Other studies showed that the brains of affected individuals are significantly smaller than unaffected controls and that the prefrontal cortex, basal ganglia, and cerebellum are differentially affected, along with reduced connectivity in white matter tracts. In addition, it has been shown that individuals diagnosed with ADHD have fewer dopaminergic receptors in the frontal lobe compared to the general population. Genome-wide associated studies reported a correlation between ADHD and variants of dopamine receptor genes DRD4 and DRD5 and transcription factor gene FOXP2. However, there are no consistent findings of neuroimaging among patients diagnosed with ADHD, and no biomarkers have been proven to date for the diagnosis of ADHD. Thus, it remains a clinical diagnosis [21–25].

3.4 Diagnostic updates

The revision of DSM diagnostic criteria in 2013 has taken into consideration the major diagnostic challenges and contributed to improving the accuracy of the ADHD diagnosis process. Notably, the adjustments addressed the increasing prevalence of ADHD among adolescents and adults and directed attention to this age group by tailoring the criteria to facilitate their assessment. The updated version re-highlighted that persistence of inattention and/or hyperactivity/impulsivity symptoms in a way that is interfering with functioning and healthy development is an essential criterion for diagnosis. All symptoms must be consistent in at least two settings to make the diagnosis. Besides, the updated version emphasized that assessment should rule out that symptoms are solely a manifestation of oppositional behavior, defiance, hostility, or failure to understand tasks or instructions.

The core symptoms of inattention and hyperactivity/impulsivity required for diagnosis remained the same. However, the more detailed description was added to address the way by which symptoms may present in older adolescents and adults (age 17 and older). In addition, the requirement of six or more symptoms in either domain to make the diagnosis was decreased to a minimum of five symptoms to make the diagnosis in older adolescents and adults. Given the potential inaccuracy in remembering ADHD symptoms from earlier ages, and the tendency of inattentive symptoms to emerge later in life, the age threshold for the onset of ADHD symptoms was adjusted from 7 to 12 years of age. This increases the chance of diagnosis in older adolescents and adults experiencing impairment.

The classification of ADHD into the three categories of predominantly inattentive, predominantly hyperactive/impulsive, or combined categories remains the same, apart from labeling subtypes as "presentations" instead of "types." This change reflects that symptomatology at the time of diagnosis may change with age and development. The updated manual requires specification of partial remission if present. This is applicable if the full criteria were previously met, and fewer of the criteria have been met in the last 6 months, but the symptoms continue to cause social, academic, and/or functional impairment. Moreover, the severity of the diagnosis should be specified as mild, moderate, or severe. Last, the updated criteria allow the diagnosis of ADHD along with autism spectrum disorder (ASD) if applicable, in contrast to the previous version [13, 26–27].

Due to the increasing frequency of ADHD, the most common condition among the category of neurodevelopmental disorders, which was newly added to the latest DSM manual, health care providers should be familiar with the process of evaluation and diagnosis of ADHD. In addition, public health campaigns should aim at raising awareness of the society, including caregivers and teachers, about concerns for which they should seek medical attention for evaluation of possible ADHD. The evaluation process should focus on detailed history taking to elicit risk factors, symptoms with their setting and frequency, degree of impairment, and symptoms of differential diagnoses or potential comorbidities. DSM-5-based rating scales can help in gathering information from different settings [28].

4. Comorbidities

4.1 Examples and implications

ADHD is a multifaceted condition that carries challenges in terms of diagnosis and treatment for different reasons. One of the main challenging aspects of ADHD is that it is frequently associated with other comorbidities that may complicate the clinical presentation, impairments, and the management plan. In many cases, the comorbidities can result from late diagnosis or improper management of ADHD as the primary problem. It has been highlighted in the literature that ADHD can be associated with other neurodevelopmental disorders, including learning disabilities, along with internalizing and externalizing psychiatric disorders. Estimates show that around 60% of children diagnosed with ADHD are affected by one or more comorbidities that often continue into adulthood [29]. Risk factors for having ADHD with comorbidities include higher severity of symptoms and a combined ADHD presentation.

4.2 Neurodevelopmental comorbidities

Neurodevelopmental disorders that have been shown to be associated with ADHD include autism spectrum disorder, learning disabilities, and tics disorder. A study from the United States showed that 59% of children diagnosed with autism spectrum disorder have comorbid ADHD. In addition, it has been shown that children with autism and comorbid ADHD have more severe symptoms across all domains of assessment and increased severity of sleep-related difficulties [30]. Although the clinical picture of autism and ADHD may overlap, Mayes et al. discussed the discriminating symptoms that help differentiate each condition from the other. For example, children with ASD are characterized by rare involvement in social interaction and communication, besides having unique motor and verbal behaviors, whereas the similar picture of ADHD is more about being easily distracted, unable to pay attention, and having difficulty sustaining mental effort. In addition, "the rapid letter naming task" was reported as a tool that showed a significant difference between the two conditions, as children with ASD showed better performance than children with ADHD but required more time. Genetic and environmental links, such as preterm delivery, have been reported between the conditions of ADHD and ASD [31, 32].

Besides autism spectrum disorder, several studies have pointed to the association of ADHD with learning disabilities, with a rate of 20–60%. A learning disability in writing was twice as prevalent compared to learning disabilities in reading, math, or spelling. Expectedly, the presence of one condition complicates the other since patients with ADHD have more severe learning disabilities, and patients with learning disabilities have more severe attention problems [30, 31, 33]. Other neurodevelopmental disorders that showed association with ADHD are tic disorders. ADHD was associated with Tourette's syndrome in around 55% of the cases. Notably, ADHD was associated with earlier diagnosis of the syndrome with a higher chance of associated difficulties such as anger management, insomnia, learning difficulties, obsessive-compulsive disorder, oppositional defiant disorder, mood disorder, and self-injurious behavior [29, 34].

4.3 Psychiatric comorbidities

In terms of psychiatric comorbidities, common comorbidities with ADHD can be classified into internalizing disorders such as depressive disorders, bipolar disorder, and anxiety disorders, along with externalizing disorders such as conduct disorder, oppositional defiant disorder, disruptive mood dysregulation disorder, and intermittent explosive disorder. Major depression was found to be five times higher in patients diagnosed with ADHD. It has been found that depressive symptoms appear later in the course of ADHD and are mostly an outcome of ADHD-related academic, social and/or occupational impairments along with negative, unsupportive environmental circumstances. Co-occurrence of bipolar disorder and ADHD results in poorer global function, increased symptom severity, and a higher chance of additional comorbidities. Similarly, the comorbidity of ADHD with anxiety has been shown to increase attentional difficulties and decrease the levels of social competence. Around 15–35% of ADHD patients experience anxiety symptoms [29, 35].

Oppositional defiant disorder and conduct disorder, along with the new entities of disruptive mood dysregulation disorder and intermittent explosive disorder, have also been found to coexist with ADHD. This can be attributed to the shared genetic origin between the conditions. Studies highlighted that the correlation increases with age and that ADHD may exacerbate the inherent externalizing tendencies. The co-occurrence is more common among boys than girls. Around 30–50% of children with ADHD fulfill the criteria for conduct disorder or oppositional defiant disorder. Risk factors of developing externalizing disorders with ADHD include neuropsychological dysfunction, early aggressive behavior and adverse family conditions. Co-existence of ADHD with externalizing disorder magnifies the functional impairment. It increases the rate of academic problems, engagement in drug abuse, and criminal behaviors, along with developing antisocial personality disorder into adulthood. Disruptive mood dysregulation disorder seems to offer an alternative description for the presence of oppositional defiant disorder or conduct disorder alongside either anxiety or ADHD. Symptoms, such as aggression, anger, and impulsivity, are also observed in intermittent explosive disorder, with a high rate of comorbidity [29, 36].

5. Management

5.1 Main pillars

The field of ADHD management modalities has undergone significant development over the past decade. Research studies, including clinical trials, have shown promising results in different domains. Therapeutic options can be classified into non-pharmacological and pharmacological modalities. Most studies focused on non-pharmacological management, which is being continuously enhanced to decrease the reliance on medications. It includes behavioral therapies, training on social skills, sleep and physical therapy interventions, meditation, devices, and hypnotherapy. Around 20% of the studies discussed the role of pharmacological therapy, which remains the mainstay of ADHD treatment. It includes Food and Drug Administration (FDA)-approved medications for ADHD, namely central nervous system stimulants, selective noradrenaline reuptake inhibitors, and alpha-2 adrenergic receptor agonists, along with other with other options that are not yet approved by the FDA for the treatment of ADHD like other antidepressants and atypical antipsychotics [37].

The bottom line is that ADHD requires a multimodal management approach that is based on multidisciplinary team input to address the several aspects of the condition, the potential comorbidities or side effects of medications. Considering the multidimensional nature of the condition, the first step of management should be a planning process between the patient, caregivers, and health care team to discuss the multimodal treatment in light of the individualized psychological, social, behavioral, academic, and occupational needs. The plan of therapeutic intervention should take into account the severity of symptoms and impairments, presence of comorbidities and their impact, resilience, and protective factors, along with the goals of the patient and caregivers. Advantages and disadvantages of each treatment modality should be clearly discussed according to the latest evidence. Similar meetings should be regularly scheduled through the treatment process to discuss the progress. The aforementioned systemic multimodal approach advocates an adaptive way of management that respects individual needs and increases the chance of success [38].

5.2 Pharmacological therapies

Unlike other psychiatric disorders, where psychosocial therapy is considered the cornerstone of management, it has been shown that medicinal treatment remains the essential component of ADHD management. Psychotherapy can be very effective if used along with medications. However, there is substantial evidence suggesting that medication management alone, without therapy, is the most effective approach [37, 38]. Pharmacological therapies for ADHD are divided into stimulant and non-stimulant medications. Stimulants are further divided into amphetamines and methylphenidate. Both types act by blocking the reuptake of dopamine at the presynaptic and postsynaptic membranes, to increase its effect. Amphetamines also release dopamine. Stimulant medications are effective in the majority of patients. There are different formulations that are classified according to their pharmacodynamic properties into immediate release and extended release formulations. Initial weekly to monthly follow-up is recommended for dosing adjustment based on clinical response [39, 40].

Adverse effects include hypertension as well as decreased appetite and sleep. Although, use of stimulants carries a risk of dependency, it has been shown that they decrease the lifetime risk of substance use that is associated with ADHD. The concern regarding stimulant use with epilepsy is no longer valid since they are deemed safe according to the latest evidence. However, they can increase tics in the case of tic disorders. This can be controlled by adding alpha agonists [16, 41].

Non-stimulant medications include antidepressants and alpha agonists. The best known antidepressant medications approved to treat ADHD is atomoxetine and the novel drug viloxazine, which works as a selective norepinephrine reuptake inhibitor. It is often used in patients who do not tolerate the side effects of stimulants or have comorbid anxiety. Other non-approved antidepressants include bupropion, which targets dopamine and norepinephrine, and tricyclic antidepressants, which target norepinephrine. In addition, alpha agonists such as clonidine and guanfacine have shown efficacy in the treatment of ADHD. However, their use is limited by potential side effects like low blood pressure, sedation, and dizziness [16, 37].

5.3 Non-pharmacological therapies

Management of ADHD should include counseling and provision of psycho-education for the patient and caregivers *via* organized programs that aim at achieving short-term and long-term goals. Several studies, including high-quality randomized controlled trials, showed widely divergent conclusions on the efficacy of psycho-social treatments in the management of ADHD, but it can be very effective if used with medications, and it is necessary to address psychosocial impairments resulting from ADHD. The modalities recommended in the management of ADHD are mainly the following: Behavior management interventions *via* caregiver training, classroom interventions and peer-based interventions, training interventions *via* cognitive behavioral therapy, cognitive training, organizational skills training and neurofeedback using electroencephalography or functional brain imaging, as well as physiological treatments like physical therapy. Other suggested non-pharmacological modalities include forms of mind-body interventions such as meditation, Yoga, mindfulness exercises, and hypnotherapy. In terms of dietary interventions, no specific diet or herbs have been shown to improve ADHD symptoms. Moreover, trigeminal nerve stimulation is the first non-pharmacological device-based treatment that was approved by the FDA for the management of ADHD in 2019. It is a noninvasive, minimal-risk modality that generates low-level electrical impulses that decrease hyperactivity [42, 43].

6. Impacts and complications

The impairments associated with ADHD symptoms and potential comorbidities can exert lifelong multidimensional impacts on the affected individuals, increasing their likelihood of experiencing negative outcomes.

6.1 Impacts on children and adolescents

In terms of health risks, ADHD has been linked to increased emergency department visits, anxiety, depression, self-harm, poor sleep, substance use disorder, as well as engagement in risky sexual behaviors [44]. Moreover, it has been shown to increase the risk of other conditions, such as obesity, binge eating, diabetes, and coronary artery disease.

French and Colleagues also discussed the several impairments associated with ADHD in their umbrella review. They reported that 16 reviews investigated the various forms of addiction associated with ADHD, eight papers highlighted the risk of suicide and self-harm, eight reviewed looked at risk of mood and personality disorders and affection of self-esteem with resultant impairments of social functioning and communication, four reviews highlighted the association with eating disorders, and 51 reviews discussed the effect of ADHD on physical health showing negative impacts on sleep, weight, oral health, risk of accidents, and injuries, along with risk of other diseases such as celiac disease, asthma, vision impairment, chronic pain, restless leg syndrome, diabetes, cardiovascular diseases, allergies, and other neurodegenerative diseases. These risks are associated with a significant reduction in quality of life.

In addition, it has several negative impacts on academic performance. For instance, it is associated with increased use of school-based services, increased rates of detention and expulsion, and decreased rates of high-school graduation or post-secondary education. Besides the deleterious effect on academic achievements, ADHD adversely impact social life and effective social functioning. It results in poor social relationships and peer interaction and increases the risk of offending and criminality [45].

6.2 Impacts on adults

If left unmanaged, ADHD can continue to cause considerable psychological, functional, educational, social, and economic challenges into adulthood that negatively affect overall quality of life. In terms of social impairment, adults with ADHD find significant difficulties in managing peer relationships or maintaining good-quality intimate relationships. The negative social impact extends into parenting skills, which also exert negative effects on children of parents with ADHD. In addition, ADHD continues to have long-term, pervasive negative educational outcomes. Some studies postulated that symptoms of inattention, rather than hyperactivity/impulsivity, may have a greater impact on measures of academic achievement [46]. Furthermore, ADHD has been consistently associated with decreased work and financial security. Evidence has consistently shown that employed adults with ADHD tend to have lower work performance, both in terms of quality and quantity. This is associated with significantly impaired life satisfaction [47]. Adults with ADHD are also at higher risk of accidents and unintentional injuries, poor sleep, substance use, and abuse, risky sexual behaviors and criminality. All aforementioned factors can contribute to higher rates of morbidity and mortality, along with diminished quality of life [48, 49].

7. Conclusion

ADHD is a prevalent neurodevelopmental disorder that significantly impacts individuals across different age groups. The diagnosis is mainly based on clinical evaluation, in Ref. to DSM-5 criteria, along with ruling out medical mimics and screening for common psychiatric or neurodevelopmental comorbidities that need to be addressed to ensure effective management. Management of ADHD typically includes a combination of pharmacological treatments and behavioral therapies and should be tailored to individual needs in order to improve functioning and decrease the multidimensional impact of the condition. It is a complex, multifaceted lifelong condition that calls for a similarly designed multimodal approach. Healthcare teams should work with patients and caregivers, aiming at early diagnosis and systemic management that adapts to different life stages and transition periods to improve quality of life. ADHD continues to be a rich area for research as it requires ongoing updates on diagnosis and management in different age groups.

Acknowledgements

We would like to acknowledge the institutional support and resources that contributed to the completion of this chapter.

Conflict of interest

The authors declare no conflict of interest.

DOI: http://dx.doi.org/10.5772/intechopen.1010652

Nomenclature

The Diagnostic and Statistical Manual of Mental Disorders (DSM)-5th edition (DSM-5): A comprehensive classification system published by the American Psychiatric Association. It provides standardized criteria for diagnosing mental health disorders, including their symptoms, diagnostic features and other relevant information. The DSM-5 is used to assess, diagnose and treat individuals with mental health conditions. The DSM-5 includes various categories of disorders, such as mood disorders, psychotic disorders, neurodevelopmental disorders and more, and it is frequently updated to reflect new research, clinical practices, and evolving understanding of mental health.

Other declarations

The authors have no other declarations.

Author details

Madeeha Kamal* and Khoulod Mohamed
Sidra Medicine, Doha, Qatar

*Address all correspondence to: mkamal1@sidra.org

References

[1] Wolraich ML, Chan E, Froehlich T, Lynch RL, Bax A, Redwine ST, et al. ADHD diagnosis and treatment guidelines: A historical perspective. Pediatrics. 2019;**144**(4):e20191682

[2] Felt BT, Biermann B, Christner JG, Kochhar P, Harrison RV. Diagnosis and management of ADHD in children. American Family Physician. 2014;**90**(7):456-464

[3] Ayano G, Demelash S, Gizachew Y, Tsegay L, Alati R. The global prevalence of attention deficit hyperactivity disorder in children and adolescents: An umbrella review of meta-analyses. Journal of Affective Disorders. 2023;**339**:860-866

[4] Al-Wardat M, Etoom M, Almhdawi KA, Hawamdeh Z, Khader Y. Prevalence of attention-deficit hyperactivity disorder in children, adolescents and adults in the Middle East and North Africa region: A systematic review and meta-analysis. BMJ Open. 2024;**14**(1):e078849

[5] Bradshaw LG, Kamal M. Prevalence of ADHD in Qatari school-age children. Journal of Attention Disorders. 2014;**21**(5):442-449

[6] Mowlem FD, Rosenqvist MA, Martin J, Lichtenstein P, Asherson P, Larsson H. Sex differences in predicting ADHD clinical diagnosis and pharmacological treatment. European Child & Adolescent Psychiatry. 2019;**28**(4):481-489

[7] Taylor MJ, Lichtenstein P, Larsson H, Anckarsäter H, Greven CU, Ronald A. Is there a female protective effect against attention-deficit/hyperactivity disorder? Evidence from two representative twin samples. Journal of the American Academy of Child and Adolescent Psychiatry. 2016;**55**(6):504-512.e2

[8] Young S, Adamo N, Ásgeirsdóttir BB, Branney P, Beckett M, Colley W, et al. Females with ADHD: An expert consensus statement taking a lifespan approach providing guidance for the identification and treatment of attention-deficit/hyperactivity disorder in girls and women. BMC Psychiatry. 2020;**20**(1):404

[9] Wilens TE, Biederman J, Faraone SV, Martelon M, Westerberg D, Spencer TJ. Presenting ADHD symptoms, subtypes, and comorbid disorders in clinically referred adults with ADHD. The Journal of Clinical Psychiatry. 2009;**70**(11):1557-1562

[10] Vos M, Hartman CA. The decreasing prevalence of ADHD across the adult lifespan confirmed. Journal of Global Health. 2022;**12**:03024

[11] Sibley MH, Swanson JM, Arnold LE, Hechtman LT, Owens EB, Stehli A, et al. Defining ADHD symptom persistence in adulthood: Optimizing sensitivity and specificity. Journal of Child Psychology and Psychiatry. 2017;**58**(6):655-662

[12] Caye A, Swanson J, Thapar A, Sibley M, Arseneault L, Hechtman L, et al. Life span studies of ADHD-conceptual challenges and predictors of persistence and outcome. Current Psychiatry Reports. 2016;**18**(12):111

[13] Substance Abuse and Mental Health Services Administration. Table 7, DSM-IV to DSM-5 Attention-Deficit/Hyperactivity Disorder Comparison [Internet]. Nih.gov. Substance Abuse and Mental Health Services Administration (US); 2016. Available from: https://www.

ncbi.nlm.nih.gov/books/NBK519712/table/ch3.t3/

[14] Gilligan RM. Supporting learners with attention deficit hyperactivity disorder: A professional development curriculum for elementary teachers [dissertation]. California (USA): University of Southern California; 2020

[15] Pujalte GGA, Narducci DM, Smith MS, King R, Logan K, Callender SS, et al. Athletes with attention-deficit/hyperactivity disorder: Position statement of the American medical Society for Sports Medicine. Clinical Journal of Sport Medicine. 2023;**33**(3):195-208

[16] Magnus W, Anilkumar AC, Shaban K. Attention deficit hyperactivity disorder. In: StatPearls [Internet]. Treasure Island (FL): StatPearls Publishing; 2023. p. 2025

[17] Harrison AG, Nay S, Armstrong IT. Diagnostic accuracy of the Conners' adult ADHD rating scale in a postsecondary population. Journal of Attention Disorders. 2019;**23**(14):1829-1837

[18] Kakubo SM, Mendez M, Silveira JD, Maringolo L, Nitta C, Silveira DXD, et al. Translation and validation of the Brown attention-deficit disorder scale for use in Brazil: Identifying cases of attention-deficit/hyperactivity disorder among samples of substance users and non-users. Cross-cultural validation study. São Paulo Medical Journal. 2018;**136**(2):157-164

[19] Pearl PL, Weiss RE, Stein MA. Medical mimics. Medical and neurological conditions simulating ADHD. Annals of the New York Academy of Sciences. 2001;**931**:97-112

[20] Sadek J. Attention deficit hyperactivity disorder misdiagnosis: Why medical evaluation should be a part of ADHD assessment. Brain Sciences. 2023;**13**(11):1522

[21] Albaugh MD, Hudziak JJ, Ing A, Chaarani B, Barker E, Jia T, et al. White matter microstructure is associated with hyperactive/inattentive symptomatology and polygenic risk for attention-deficit/hyperactivity disorder in a population-based sample of adolescents. Neuropsychopharmacology. 2019;**44**(9):1597-1603

[22] Curatolo P, D'Agati E, Moavero R. The neurobiological basis of ADHD. Italian Journal of Pediatrics. 2010;**36**(1):79. DOI: 10.1186/1824-7288-36-79

[23] Hayashi W, Iwanami A. Biological mechanisms of ADHD. Brain and Nerve. 2018;**70**(11):1265-1277

[24] Brennan AR, Arnsten AF. Neuronal mechanisms underlying attention deficit hyperactivity disorder: The influence of arousal on prefrontal cortical function. Annals of the New York Academy of Sciences. 2008;**1129**:236-245

[25] Cabral MDI, Liu S, Soares N. Attention-deficit/hyperactivity disorder: Diagnostic criteria, epidemiology, risk factors and evaluation in youth. Translational Pediatrics. 2020;**9**(Suppl. 1):S104-S113

[26] Epstein JN, Loren RE. Changes in the definition of ADHD in DSM-5: Subtle but important. Neuropsychiatry (London). 2013;**3**(5):455-458

[27] Koutsoklenis A, Honkasilta J. ADHD in the DSM-5-TR: What has changed and what has not. Frontiers in Psychiatry. 2023;**13**:1064141

[28] Eom TH, Kim YH. Clinical practice guidelines for attention-deficit/

hyperactivity disorder: Recent updates. Clinical and Experimental Pediatrics. 2024;**67**(1):26-34

[29] Gnanavel S, Sharma P, Kaushal P, Hussain S. Attention deficit hyperactivity disorder and comorbidity: A review of literature. World Journal of Clinical Cases. 2019;**7**(17):2420-2426

[30] Jogia J, Sharif AH, Nawaz FA, Khan AR, Alawami RH, Aljanahi MA, et al. Comorbidities associated with attention-deficit/hyperactivity disorder in children and adolescents at a tertiary care setting. Global Pediatric Health. 2022;**9**:2333794X221076607

[31] Mayes SD, Calhoun SL, Crowell EW. Learning disabilities and ADHD: Overlapping spectrum disorders. Journal of Learning Disabilities. 2000;**33**:417-424

[32] Al Ghamdi K, AlMusailhi J. Attention-deficit hyperactivity disorder and autism spectrum disorder: Towards better diagnosis and management. Medical Archives. 2024;**78**(2):159-163

[33] Czamara D, Tiesler CM, Kohlböck G, Berdel D, Hoffmann B, Bauer CP, et al. Children with ADHD symptoms have a higher risk for reading, spelling and math difficulties in the GINIplus and LISAplus cohort studies. PLoS One. 2013;**8**(5):e63859

[34] Spencer T, Biederman J, Wilens T. Attention-deficit/hyperactivity disorder and comorbidity. Pediatric Clinics of North America. 1999;**46**:915-927

[35] Sandstrom A, Perroud N, Alda M, Uher R, Pavlova B. Prevalence of attention-deficit/hyperactivity disorder in people with mood disorders: A systematic review and meta-analysis. Acta Psychiatrica Scandinavica. 2021;**143**(5):380-391

[36] Kuja-Halkola R, Lichtenstein P, D'Onofrio BM, Larsson H. Codevelopment of ADHD and externalizing behavior from childhood to adulthood. Journal of Child Psychology and Psychiatry. 2015;**56**(6):640-647

[37] Nazarova VA, Sokolov AV, Chubarev VN, Tarasov VV, Schiöth HB. Treatment of ADHD: Drugs, psychological therapies, devices, complementary and alternative methods as well as the trends in clinical trials. Frontiers in Pharmacology. 2022;**13**:1066988

[38] Drechsler R, Brem S, Brandeis D, Grünblatt E, Berger G, Walitza S. ADHD: Current concepts and treatments in children and adolescents. Neuropediatrics. 2020;**51**(5):315-335

[39] Geffen J, Forster K. Treatment of adult ADHD: A clinical perspective. Therapeutic Advances in Psychopharmacology. 2018;**8**(1):25-32

[40] Ching C, Eslick GD, Poulton AS. Evaluation of methylphenidate safety and maximum-dose titration rationale in attention-deficit/hyperactivity disorder: A meta-analysis. JAMA Pediatrics. 2019;**173**(7):630-639

[41] Advokat C, Scheithauer M. Attention-deficit hyperactivity disorder (ADHD) stimulant medications as cognitive enhancers. Frontiers in Neuroscience. 2013;**7**:82

[42] Shrestha M, Lautenschleger J, Soares N. Non-pharmacologic management of attention-deficit/hyperactivity disorder in children and adolescents: A review. Translational Pediatrics. 2020;**9**(Suppl. 1):S114-S124

[43] Loo SK, Salgari GC, Ellis A, Cowen J, Dillon A, McGough JJ. Trigeminal nerve stimulation for attention-deficit/hyperactivity disorder: Cognitive and electroencephalographic predictors

of treatment response. Journal of the American Academy of Child and Adolescent Psychiatry. 2021;**60**(7):856-864.e1

[44] Schoenfelder EN, Kollins SH. Topical review: ADHD and health-risk behaviors: Toward prevention and health promotion. Journal of Pediatric Psychology. Aug 2016;**41**(7):735-740

[45] French B, Nalbant G, Wright H, Sayal K, Daley D, Groom MJ, et al. The impacts associated with having ADHD: An umbrella review. Frontiers in Psychiatry. 2024;**15**:1343314

[46] Kosheleff AR, Mason O, Jain R, Koch J, Rubin J. Functional impairments associated with ADHD in adulthood and the impact of pharmacological treatment. Journal of Attention Disorders. 2023;**27**(7):669-697

[47] Safren SA, Sprich SE, Cooper-Vince CE, Knouse LE, Lerner JA. Life impairments in adults with medication-treated ADHD. Journal of Attention Disorders. 2010;**13**(5):524-531

[48] Quintero J, Morales I, Vera R, Zuluaga P, Fernández A. The impact of adult ADHD in the quality of life profile. Journal of Attention Disorders. 2019;**23**(9):1007-1016

[49] Harpin VA. The effect of ADHD on the life of an individual, their family, and community from preschool to adult life. Archives of Disease in Childhood. 2005;**90**(Suppl. 1):i2-i7

Chapter 7

The Role of Artificial Intelligence in ADHD Diagnosis and Treatment: A New Frontier in Neurotechnology

Selman Yildirim

Abstract

Recent advancements in artificial intelligence (AI) are opening new frontiers in the diagnosis and treatment of Attention Deficit Hyperactivity Disorder (ADHD). AI-powered technologies such as machine learning, natural language processing, and predictive analytics have the potential to enhance ADHD assessment by analyzing complex patterns in large datasets, such as neuroimaging, genetic information, and behavioral data. These technologies can support clinicians in early diagnosis and personalized treatment planning. Furthermore, AI applications are increasingly being explored in the context of behavioral therapies and neurostimulation techniques, such as transcranial magnetic stimulation (TMS) and transcranial direct current stimulation (tDCS), to optimize ADHD interventions. This chapter will explore the integration of AI in ADHD care, discussing its benefits, challenges, and future implications for improving ADHD management.

Keywords: ADHD, AI, neurotechnology, treatment, innovation

1. Introduction

Attention-Deficit/Hyperactivity Disorder (ADHD) is a neurodevelopmental condition marked by inattention, impulsivity, and hyperactivity, with origins in complex genetic, neurobiological, and environmental interactions [1, 2]. It often begins in childhood and can persist into adulthood, affecting emotional regulation and social functioning [1]. Prevalence rates vary globally—estimated at 5–7% in children and about 2.8% in adults—shaped by cultural, socioeconomic, and methodological factors [2–6]. ADHD significantly impacts academic performance, peer relationships, and co-occurs with other psychiatric conditions, contributing to long-term social and economic burdens [7, 8]. Early, comprehensive intervention is essential to improve outcomes and reduce societal costs [9, 10].

The diagnosis and treatment of ADHD involve significant challenges due to symptom overlap with other neurodevelopmental conditions, particularly Autism Spectrum Disorder (ASD), leading to diagnostic uncertainty, especially in cases of comorbidity [11, 12]. These challenges are further amplified during times of crisis, such as the COVID-19 pandemic, when external stressors and disruptions in routine—particularly within educational settings—can intensify symptom presentation and complicate differential diagnosis [13, 14]. Variations in diagnostic criteria across regions further contribute to inconsistencies, resulting in both over- and underdiagnosis in different jurisdictions [15]. Accurate diagnosis is especially difficult in populations with intellectual disabilities, where symptoms may present atypically, and subjective clinical judgments can lead to misdiagnosis unless supported by standardized tools [16]. In adults, overlapping symptoms with conditions such as depression can obscure underlying ADHD, complicating diagnosis [17]. Treatment outcomes depend heavily on accurate diagnosis and recognition of comorbidities, requiring a combined pharmacological and psychosocial approach [18, 19]. Additionally, stigma within primary care settings and shifting symptom presentation across the lifespan underscore the need for flexible, informed, and individualized care strategies [18, 20].

Just as the diagnosis and treatment of complex psychiatric conditions like ADHD involve multifaceted challenges, another major transformation is unfolding in modern medicine: the rise of artificial intelligence (AI). While AI holds tremendous potential to enhance the accuracy, efficiency, and accessibility of healthcare, its integration into clinical practice requires careful ethical and regulatory consideration. Through technologies such as deep learning, natural language processing, and machine learning, AI is being applied in various domains—including medical imaging and predictive analytics—with diagnostic performance often comparable to human experts [21–23]. However, concerns remain regarding the limited clinical validation of many AI tools, issues of algorithmic transparency, and patient data privacy [24, 25]. Ethical challenges—such as algorithmic bias, accountability, and the role of human oversight—also shape public perception and acceptance of AI in medicine [26, 27]. Furthermore, disparities in AI access across populations raise the risk of exacerbating existing healthcare inequalities, underscoring the importance of ensuring equitable deployment [27]. Therefore, for AI to be successfully and fairly integrated into healthcare systems, ongoing research, transparent regulations, and ethical frameworks are essential.

Building on the broader discussion of artificial intelligence in medicine, its application in the management of ADHD presents a rapidly advancing frontier. AI-driven innovations are not only enhancing diagnostic precision but also enabling personalized treatments and adaptive educational strategies that are particularly beneficial in neurodevelopmental disorders like ADHD.

AI technologies significantly improve diagnostic accuracy by analyzing neuroimaging data and behavioral patterns using advanced machine learning models such as temporal convolutional networks, which have shown promising results in identifying ADHD-related brain connectivity profiles [28, 29]. Moreover, AI enables the development of individualized treatment and educational plans by adjusting in real time to a patient's specific learning style and therapeutic needs, thereby improving engagement and outcomes [30, 31]. AI-powered telehealth tools further enhance treatment adherence and access to care, especially in underserved communities, by offering continuous monitoring and timely feedback [32, 33]. In addition, interactive AI applications—including serious video games and virtual reality tools—are gaining traction as engaging methods to enhance cognitive functioning and attention in children with ADHD [34, 35]. AI also contributes to ADHD research by analyzing extensive behavioral and neurophysiological datasets, allowing for the identification of personalized treatment responses, while developments in explainable AI ensure clinical transparency and trust in AI-generated outputs [36]. Collectively, these innovations suggest that AI holds transformative potential for ADHD care, despite ongoing challenges related to ethics, validation, and implementation.

2. Difficulties in diagnosing ADHD

The clinical diagnosis of ADHD involves considerable subjectivity due to its reliance on observational data, self-report measures, and DSM criteria. Observational methods, such as clinician interviews and behavior assessments, can be inconsistent and influenced by practitioner biases [37]. Many clinicians fail to use standardized rating scales or adhere strictly to DSM guidelines, leading to variable diagnostic practices [38]. Self-report tools like the ADHD Rating Scale and ACDS are prone to over- or under-reporting, influenced by stigma and symptom misinterpretation [39]. Moreover, discrepancies often exist between subjective reports and objective neuropsychological assessments, risking misdiagnosis [40]. The DSM criteria themselves have evolved over time, but concerns remain regarding their temporal stability and the impact of revisions on diagnosis rates [41]. Additionally, racial and ethnic disparities suggest that minority children may be underdiagnosed due to systemic and clinician biases, despite no actual difference in ADHD prevalence [42]. This highlights the need for cultural competence in diagnostic practices [43]. Emerging technologies, including AI applications analyzing neuroimaging and behavioral data, offer potential for improving diagnostic objectivity, though these innovations are not yet ready for widespread clinical use [29].

Diagnosing ADHD is often complicated by comorbid conditions such as anxiety, depression, cognitive disengagement syndrome, and ASD, which can obscure the clinical picture and contribute to under- or misdiagnosis. These comorbidities frequently share overlapping symptoms with ADHD, such as inattention, impulsivity, and emotional dysregulation, making differential diagnosis challenging [11, 44, 45]. Anxiety and depression are especially common among individuals with ADHD and can alter symptom presentation and treatment responses—particularly to stimulant medications [46, 47]. Comorbid ASD in children can also impact healthcare delivery, further obscuring ADHD symptoms and leading caregivers and patients to misattribute behaviors [48, 49]. ADHD subtypes also differ in comorbidity patterns, with the inattentive subtype showing a higher prevalence of anxiety disorders. The presence of comorbid conditions has implications for diagnosis, treatment adherence, and overall health-related quality of life. Therefore, accurate diagnosis requires a comprehensive, multi-dimensional evaluation that accounts for overlapping symptoms and co-occurring disorders. Improved clinician training and diagnostic tools are essential for enhancing outcomes [50, 51].

Delays in ADHD diagnosis—especially among adults—are common and can lead to prolonged functional impairments and increased risk of comorbid conditions such as major depressive disorder [52, 53]. One Canadian study found that one-third of adult referrals experienced delays of over 3 months [52]. These delays are often due to limited awareness of adult ADHD, insufficient screening tools, and the masking effects of comorbid disorders like anxiety and depression [54, 55]. Overdiagnosis, on the other hand, stems from the subjective nature of ADHD symptoms and overreliance on behavioral checklists such as the SNAP or IOWA scales, which can lead to false positives if not supplemented with thorough clinical evaluation [56]. Cultural and systemic factors, including pressure from educators or parents to access academic support, can further contribute to inflated diagnosis rates. Additionally, the DSM criteria—originally designed for children—may not accurately reflect adult symptom presentations, leading to both under- and overdiagnosis in different cases [57]. Delayed diagnosis can result in more severe presentations and missed treatment opportunities, while overdiagnosis can lead to inappropriate treatment and stigma. Both contribute to diagnostic uncertainty and may reduce trust in mental health services [58]. Improving ADHD diagnosis requires standardized protocols, greater awareness of adult ADHD, and attention to comorbidities. Ongoing education for clinicians is essential to reduce both diagnostic delays and overdiagnosis.

Given these challenges in ADHD diagnosis—whether due to delays, overdiagnosis, or limitations in assessment tools—it becomes clear that neuropsychological testing alone cannot address the full complexity of identifying ADHD accurately. Neuropsychological tests have significant limitations in diagnosing Attention-Deficit/Hyperactivity Disorder (ADHD), as they often fail to capture the disorder's full complexity. While these assessments measure specific cognitive functions (e.g., attention, executive functioning), they may overlook key ADHD symptoms such as emotional dysregulation and impulsivity, leading to potential false negatives [59]. Additionally, symptom overlap with other conditions (e.g., anxiety, learning disabilities) complicates differential diagnosis, as impairments in attention are not unique to ADHD [60]. Test performance can also be influenced by situational factors like motivation and emotional state, raising concerns about reliability [61]. Furthermore, neuropsychological results often lack strong predictive validity for real-world functioning, meaning they may not accurately reflect academic or occupational challenges [62]. Overreliance on these tests risks misdiagnosis, particularly when external pressures (e.g., educational demands) incentivize quick diagnoses without comprehensive evaluation [63, 64]. Lastly, while executive function deficits are central to ADHD, lab-based tests may not fully translate to real-life impairments, limiting their ecological validity [62, 65]. Given these limitations, a multimodal approach—incorporating behavioral observations, parent/teacher reports, and longitudinal assessments—is crucial for an accurate ADHD diagnosis [61–63].

3. Fundamentals of artificial intelligence and its relationship with ADHD

Artificial Intelligence (AI), Machine Learning (ML), and Deep Learning (DL) are transformative technologies that enhance human cognitive functions, with significant applications in healthcare, finance, and data analysis. AI enables machines to perform complex tasks such as reasoning, learning, and decision-making, proving particularly valuable in clinical diagnostics and medical imaging analysis for conditions like epilepsy [66, 67]. ML, a subset of AI, leverages algorithms to identify patterns in data, improving predictive accuracy for patient outcomes—such as readmission risks in adrenal insufficiency—though its efficacy depends on data quality and sample size [66, 68]. DL, a specialized ML approach using deep neural networks, excels in processing unstructured data like medical images, with convolutional neural networks (CNNs) achieving high accuracy in image analysis [67, 69]. Despite their potential, challenges like the need for large labeled datasets and model generalization persist [66, 70]. Ongoing advancements in these fields promise to revolutionize healthcare and beyond.

Artificial Intelligence (AI) systems are transforming ADHD diagnosis by leveraging machine learning (ML) and deep learning (DL) to analyze multimodal data, improving accuracy and efficiency. Studies highlight the use of neuroimaging (MRI, EEG) to identify neurological ADHD markers, with ML classifiers achieving over 80% accuracy in distinguishing ADHD subtypes [71, 72]. DL models, such as CNNs, enhance diagnostic precision, reaching sensitivities of 91% in EEG-based classifications [73]. Automated algorithms integrate demographic, clinical, and neuropsychological data, achieving 81% accuracy in pediatric ADHD diagnosis [74], while multimodal approaches aid early detection in preschoolers [75]. Genetic data analysis via DL achieves 90% accuracy in linking SNPs to ADHD [76], and low-cost ML models using behavioral video data improve accessibility [36]. Explainable AI frameworks further support clinicians by clarifying diagnostic decisions, fostering trust and early intervention [36]. Overall, AI-driven tools offer objective, comprehensive ADHD assessments, enabling timely and accurate diagnoses.

Artificial Intelligence (AI) is increasingly being used by utilizing various forms of input data, including survey data, electroencephalogram (EEG) readings, functional magnetic resonance imaging (fMRI), behavioral analyses, video recordings, and electronic health records (EHR). These data types can enhance diagnostic accuracy and facilitate timely interventions.

Surveys play a crucial role in the initial identification of ADHD symptoms by collecting information from parents, teachers, and patients themselves. These reports often serve as primary evidence in the diagnostic process. AI systems can analyze large volumes of survey responses to identify patterns and correlations that may not be apparent through traditional evaluation methods. However, the specific references used in this context do not directly relate to the analysis of survey data for ADHD diagnostics, and thus, this statement should be made without citation.

Electroencephalography data are pivotal in studying the cortical processes associated with ADHD symptoms. Deep learning models, such as CNNs, have been shown to effectively differentiate children with ADHD from healthy controls using EEG signals. For instance, research indicates that deep learning architectures can achieve classification accuracies around 80% between children with ADHD and healthy controls, thereby allowing for more objective symptom identification in clinical settings [71, 73].

Functional Magnetic Resonance Imaging (fMRI) provides insights into brain function and connectivity, which are instrumental in understanding the neurobiological aspects of ADHD. Although some studies indicate that deep learning models utilizing fMRI data can classify ADHD subtypes, references indicating specific advances related to the differentiation between ADHD and other psychiatric disorders were not found in the provided citations. Therefore, any mention of increased precision in this context should either be supported by appropriate citations or omitted.

AI can analyze behavioral data collected through various means, including observational studies and formal assessments of children's interactions with tasks or peers. Machine learning algorithms can identify behavioral patterns over time that assist in identifying subtypes of ADHD. The claim that behavioral data can be derived from structured assessments and evaluated by AI systems lacks supporting references, necessitating either the citation of evidence or the removal of this statement.

The use of video recordings offers an innovative approach to observing real-life behavior in children suspected of having ADHD. AI and machine learning techniques can analyze video recordings to detect abnormal behaviors or patterns indicative of ADHD symptoms, such as impulsivity or inattentiveness. The ability of AI to identify movement patterns, gaze direction, and other non-verbal cues is supported by research, but the specific work by Lee et al. [77] discusses abnormal behaviors in the context of a robot-led screening game, which may not fully correspond to the broader application mentioned. Therefore, an accurate citation must be included, or the context should be adjusted accordingly.

The integration of EHR data can provide a comprehensive view of a patient's medical history, including previous diagnoses, treatments, and comorbid conditions. AI systems can analyze EHR data to identify patterns that correlate with the diagnosis of ADHD and to assist in treatment management. There is evidence that AI systems can leverage EHR data in this capacity, although the work by Liu et al. [78] specifically focuses on EEG applications and may not fully support claims regarding EHR, necessitating scrutiny.

In conclusion, while the utilization of diverse data types such as survey data, EEG, fMRI, behavioral analyses, video recordings, and EHR has the potential to enhance the ADHD diagnostic process through AI integration, some claims need to be explicitly supported by peer-reviewed literature to ensure accuracy. Furthermore, references that do not directly contribute to the claims made should be omitted for a clearer presentation of facts.

4. AI-based ADHD treatment approaches

Artificial Intelligence (AI) systems are increasingly employed in the treatment of Attention-Deficit/Hyperactivity Disorder (ADHD) through various innovative approaches that enhance traditional treatment modalities. These AI-driven strategies utilize technology to support therapeutic interventions and improve patient outcomes.

AI-enhanced virtual reality (VR) technologies are emerging as effective tools for managing ADHD symptoms. Recent studies have indicated that VR-based interventions can be beneficial in controlling impulsive and aggressive behaviors associated with ADHD, and they may help prevent potential delinquency among adolescents with these symptoms [79]. By immersing individuals in simulated environments that require focus and behavioral regulation, these interventions can reinforce positive coping strategies and reduce behavioral problems.

AI's role in behavioral therapy includes tailoring interventions to match the specific needs of children with ADHD. Parent-training programs facilitated by AI can guide parents in implementing effective behavioral management strategies at home. These AI-assisted programs align with national guidelines that recommend behavioral therapy as a first-line treatment for preschool-aged children with ADHD [80]. Additionally, AI can personalize these programs based on real-time feedback and progress tracking.

Machine learning algorithms can analyze clinical data to identify patterns that inform treatment approaches for ADHD [81, 82]. For instance, studies using Conners' Adult ADHD Rating Scales in combination with machine learning techniques have demonstrated promise in distinguishing between ADHD and other clinical conditions, enhancing the precision of treatment strategies [82]. By automating diagnostic classifications, AI helps ensure that patients receive treatment tailored to their specific ADHD subtype.

AI systems can utilize Electronic Health Records (EHR) data to track treatment outcomes and identify effective interventions over time. Analyzing large datasets within EHRs allows AI tools to provide insights into patterns of treatment efficacy, facilitating data-driven decision-making in clinical practices [83]. This integration enables practitioners to adapt treatment plans based on individual patient histories and responses to interventions.

AI is also being explored in conjunction with Cognitive Behavioral Therapy (CBT) to optimize treatment pathways for individuals with ADHD. Personalized AI-assisted CBT programs can enhance traditional therapeutic practices by providing tools for addressing negative thought patterns and developing coping strategies. Furthermore, studies indicate that combining VR technology with CBT techniques may enhance engagement and efficacy in treatment protocols for ADHD [84, 85].

AI applications in neuroimaging, particularly through machine learning models analyzing functional and structural MRI data, have been instrumental in identifying ADHD-related neurobiological differences. Such approaches underline the potential for personalized treatment based on neurophysiological insights [86]. AI aids in creating predictive models that classify ADHD more accurately, which can lead to more tailored therapeutic approaches.

To sum up, AI-driven methodologies in treating ADHD encompass a range of strategies, from VR and machine learning-based interventions to enhancing traditional therapeutic practices like CBT. These emerging technologies not only improve the precision of ADHD diagnosis and treatment but also offer significant prospects for personalizing care to meet the unique needs of individuals with ADHD. Continued research and development of these AI applications are essential for realizing their full potential in ADHD management.

5. Conclusion

ADHD is a complex neurodevelopmental disorder shaped by genetic, neurobiological, and environmental factors, posing significant challenges in diagnosis and treatment. Current diagnostic methods remain limited due to symptom overlap and comorbidities, but artificial intelligence (AI) offers promising solutions by analyzing neuroimaging, behavioral data, and electronic health records for more objective and personalized assessments. AI-driven tools, including telehealth platforms, virtual reality therapies, and machine learning models, enhance treatment adherence and accessibility. However, challenges such as ethical concerns, algorithmic biases, and limited clinical validation persist. To fully realize AI's potential in ADHD management, multicenter research, standardized protocols, and culturally sensitive ethical frameworks are essential. By addressing these barriers, AI-powered innovations can play a transformative role in improving the quality of life for individuals with ADHD. Continued collaboration between clinicians, researchers, and technologists will be key to advancing equitable and effective ADHD care.

Author details

Selman Yildirim
Region Blekinge Child and Adolescent Psychiatry Department, Karlskrona, Sweden

*Address all correspondence to: selmann.yildirim1@gmail.com

References

[1] Soliva JC, Carmona S, Fauquet J, Hoekzema E, Bulbena A, Hilferty J, et al. Neurobiological substrates of social cognition impairment in attention-deficit hyperactivity disorder. Annals of the New York Academy of Sciences. 2009;**1167**(1):212-220

[2] Song P, Zha M, Yang Q, Zhang Y, Li X, Rudan I. The prevalence of adult attention-deficit hyperactivity disorder: A global systematic review and meta-analysis. Journal of Global Health. 2021;**11**:04009

[3] Catalá-López F, Peiró S, Ridao M, Sanfélix-Gimeno G, Gènova-Maleras R, Catalá MA. Prevalence of attention deficit hyperactivity disorder among children and adolescents in Spain: A systematic review and meta-analysis of epidemiological studies. BMC Psychiatry. 2012;**12**(1):168

[4] He Z, Yang X, Li Y, Zhao X, Li J, Li B. Attention-deficit/hyperactivity disorder in children with epilepsy: A systematic review and meta-analysis of prevalence and risk factors. Epilepsia Open. 2024;**9**(4):1148-1165

[5] Alhraiwil NJ, Ali A, Househ MS, Al-Shehri AM, El-Metwally AA. Systematic review of the epidemiology of attention deficit hyperactivity disorder in Arab countries. Neurosciences. 2015;**20**(2):137-144

[6] Lee J, Lee SI, Lee YM, Hong YH. Prevalence of attention deficit hyperactivity disorder in girls with central precocious puberty. Journal of Attention Disorders. 2023;**27**(13):1460-1466

[7] Moulin F, Chollet A, Ramos-Quiroga JA, Bouvard M, Melchior M, Galéra C. Prevalence and psychosocial correlates of ADHD symptoms in young adulthood: A French population-based study. Journal of Attention Disorders. 2018;**22**(2):167-181

[8] Rohde LA, Biederman J, Busnello EA, Zimmermann H, Schmitz M, Martins S, et al. ADHD in a school sample of Brazilian adolescents: A study of prevalence, comorbid conditions, and impairments. Journal of the American Academy of Child and Adolescent Psychiatry. 1999;**38**(6):716-722

[9] Alqarni MM, Shati AA, Alassiry MZ, Asiri WMA, Alqahtani SS, Al Zomia AS, et al. Patterns of injuries among children diagnosed with attention deficit hyperactivity disorder in Aseer region, Southwestern Saudi Arabia. Cureus. 2021;**13**(8):e17396

[10] Mugnaini D, Masi G, Brovedani P, Chelazzi C, Matas M, Romagnoli C, et al. Teacher reports of ADHD symptoms in Italian children at the end of first grade. European Psychiatry. 2006;**21**(6):419-426

[11] Yildirim S, TB; BC; TZ. Examination of symptoms related to cognitive disengagement syndrome in a clinical cohort of school-aged children. Dusunen Adam: The Journal of Psychiatry and Neurological Sciences. 2023;**36**:201-207

[12] Malwane MI, Nguyen EB, Trejo S, Kim EY, Cucalón-Calderón JR. A delayed diagnosis of autism Spectrum disorder in the setting of complex attention deficit hyperactivity disorder. Cureus. 2022;**14**(6):e25825

[13] Yildiz N, Özen N, Özkan Kart P, Yildirim S, Karadeniz S, Bilginer Ç, et al. The impact of the COVID-19 pandemic

on the educational process of children with autism spectrum disorder and effects on the parental quality of life. Turkish Journal of Pediatric Disease. 2023;**18**(1):41-48

[14] Çilem B, Selman Y, Berire ÇY, Ercüment BSK. Changes in adolescent mental health during the covid pandemic. Minerva Pediatrics. 2021;**76**(5):652-659

[15] Al-Wardat M, Etoom M, Almhdawi KA, Hawamdeh Z, Khader Y. Prevalence of attention-deficit hyperactivity disorder in children, adolescents and adults in the Middle East and North Africa region: A systematic review and meta-analysis. BMJ Open. 2024;**14**(1):e078849

[16] Perera B, Courtenay K, Solomou S, Borakati A, Strydom A. Diagnosis of attention deficit hyperactivity disorder in intellectual disability: <scp>diagnostic and statistical manual of mental disorder V</scp> versus clinical impression. Journal of Intellectual Disability Research. 2020;**64**(3):251-257

[17] Powell V, Agha SS, Jones RB, Eyre O, Stephens A, Weavers B, et al. ADHD in adults with recurrent depression. Journal of Affective Disorders. 2021;**295**:1153-1160

[18] French B, Sayal K, Daley D. Barriers and facilitators to understanding of ADHD in primary care: A mixed-method systematic review. European Child and Adolescent Psychiatry. 2019;**28**(8):1037-1064

[19] Barbaresi WJ, Campbell L, Diekroger EA, Froehlich TE, Liu YH, O'Malley E, et al. Society for developmental and behavioral pediatrics clinical practice guideline for the assessment and treatment of children and adolescents with complex attention-deficit/hyperactivity disorder. Journal of Developmental and Behavioral Pediatrics. 2020;**41**(2S):S35-S57

[20] Asherson P, Agnew-Blais J. Annual research review: Does late-onset attention-deficit/hyperactivity disorder exist? Journal of Child Psychology and Psychiatry. 2019;**60**(4):333-352

[21] IC, - RG, - SS, - K Das, - MK. Revolutionizing innovations and impact of artificial intelligence in healthcare. International Journal for Multidisciplinary Research. 2024;**6**(3):19333

[22] Krishnan G, Singh S, Pathania M, Gosavi S, Abhishek S, Parchani A, et al. Artificial intelligence in clinical medicine: Catalyzing a sustainable global healthcare paradigm. Frontiers in Artificial Intelligence. 2023;**6**:1227091

[23] Fatima I, Grover V, Raza Khan I, Ahmad N, Yadav A. Artificial Intelligence in Medical Filed. EAI Endorsed Transactions on Pervasive Health and Technology. 2023;**9**:1-5

[24] Jeyaraman M, Balaji S, Jeyaraman N, Yadav S. Unraveling the ethical enigma: Artificial intelligence in healthcare. Cureus. 2023;**15**(8):e43262

[25] Koo TH, Zakaria AD, Ng JK, Bin LX. Systematic review of the application of artificial intelligence in healthcare and nursing care. Malaysian Journal of Medical Sciences. 2024;**31**(5):135-142

[26] Prakash S, Balaji JN, Joshi A, Surapaneni KM. Ethical conundrums in the application of artificial intelligence (AI) in healthcare—A scoping review of reviews. Journal of Personalized Medicine. 2022;**12**(11):1914

[27] Stypińska J, Franke A. AI revolution in healthcare and medicine and the

(re-)emergence of inequalities and disadvantages for ageing population. Frontiers in Sociology. 2023;7:1038854

[28] Slobodin O, Yahav I, Berger I. A machine-based prediction model of ADHD using CPT data. Frontiers in Human Neuroscience. 2020;**14**:560021

[29] Wang X, Jia Q, Liang L, Zhou W, Yang W, Mu J. Artificial intelligence in ADHD: A global perspective on research hotspots, trends and clinical applications. Frontiers in Human Neuroscience. 2025;**19**:1577585

[30] Sandipa BD, Mitratne DM, Isurika MDA, Kandanaarachchi DS, Rathnayaka SC, Tissera WW. Artificial intelligence and machine learning based approach to motivate and assist primary school ADHD children. International Research Journal of Innovations in Engineering and Technology. 2023;**07**(09):89-96

[31] Barua PD, Vicnesh J, Gururajan R, Oh SL, Palmer E, Azizan MM, et al. Artificial intelligence enabled personalised assistive tools to enhance education of children with neurodevelopmental disorders—A review. International Journal of Environmental Research and Public Health. 2022;**19**(3):1192

[32] Eltyeb EE, Gohal GA, Alhazmi NH, Hamdi S, Al Khairat LH, Shutayfi NA, et al. The efficacy of educational interventions in improving school teachers' knowledge of attention deficit hyperactivity disorder. Cureus. 2023;**15**(9):e44509

[33] Choi J, Woo S, Ferrell A. Artificial intelligence assisted telehealth for nursing: A scoping review. Journal of Telemedicine and Telecare. 2025;**31**(1):140-149

[34] Rodrigo-Yanguas M, González-Tardón C, Bella-Fernández M, Blasco-Fontecilla H. Serious video games: Angels or demons in patients with attention-deficit hyperactivity disorder? A quasi-systematic review. Frontiers in Psychiatry. 2022;**13**:798480

[35] Goharinejad S, Goharinejad S, Hajesmaeel-Gohari S, Bahaadinbeigy K. The usefulness of virtual, augmented, and mixed reality technologies in the diagnosis and treatment of attention deficit hyperactivity disorder in children: An overview of relevant studies. BMC Psychiatry. 2022;**22**(1):4

[36] Rehman A, Lin JC, Heldal I. Enhancing psychologists' understanding through explainable deep learning framework for <scp>ADHD</scp> diagnosis. Expert Systems. 2025;**42**(2):e13788

[37] Alkahtani H, Aldhyani T, Ahmed Z, Alqarni A. Developing system-based artificial intelligence models for detecting the attention deficit hyperactivity disorder. Mathematics. 2023;**11**(22):4698

[38] Rowland AS, Skipper BJ, Umbach DM, Rabiner DL, Campbell RA, Naftel AJ, et al. The prevalence of ADHD in a population-based sample. Journal of Attention Disorders. 2015;**19**(9):741-754

[39] Danielson ML, Bitsko RH, Ghandour RM, Holbrook JR, Kogan MD, Blumberg SJ. Prevalence of parent-reported ADHD diagnosis and associated treatment among U.S. Children and Adolescents, 2016. Journal of Clinical Child and Adolescent Psychology. 2018;**47**(2):199-212

[40] Moffitt TE, Houts R, Asherson P, Belsky DW, Corcoran DL, Hammerle M, et al. Is adult ADHD a childhood-onset neurodevelopmental disorder? Evidence

from a four-decade longitudinal cohort study. American Journal of Psychiatry. 2015;**172**(10):967-977

[41] Fayyad J, Sampson NA, Hwang I, Adamowski T, Aguilar-Gaxiola S, Al-Hamzawi A, et al. The descriptive epidemiology of DSM-IV adult ADHD in the World Health Organization world mental health surveys. ADHD Attention Deficit and Hyperactivity Disorders. 2017;**9**(1):47-65

[42] Cree RA, Bitsko RH, Danielson ML, Wanga V, Holbrook J, Flory K, et al. Surveillance of ADHD among children in the United States: Validity and reliability of parent report of provider diagnosis. Journal of Attention Disorders. 2023;**27**(2):111-123

[43] Coker TR, Elliott MN, Toomey SL, Schwebel DC, Cuccaro P, Tortolero Emery S, et al. Racial and ethnic disparities in ADHD diagnosis and treatment. Pediatrics. 2016;**138**(3):e2016 0407-e20160407

[44] Durand G, Arbone IS. Exploring the relationship between ADHD, its common comorbidities, and their relationship to organizational skills. PeerJ. 2022;**10**:e12836

[45] Giacobini M, Ahnemark E, Medin E, Freilich J, Andersson M, Ma Y, et al. Epidemiology, treatment patterns, comorbidities, and concomitant medication in patients with ADHD in Sweden: A registry-based study (2018-2021). Journal of Attention Disorders. 2023;**27**(12):1309-1321

[46] Mao AR, Findling RL. Comorbidities in adult attention-deficit/hyperactivity disorder: A practical guide to diagnosis in primary care. Postgraduate Medicine. 2014;**126**(5):42-51

[47] Dogan-Sander E, Strauß M. Case report: Treatment of a comorbid attention deficit hyperactivity disorder and obsessive–compulsive disorder with psychostimulants. Frontiers in Psychiatry. 2021;**12**:649833

[48] Thomas S, Lycett K, Papadopoulos N, Sciberras E, Rinehart N. Exploring behavioral sleep problems in children with ADHD and comorbid autism Spectrum disorder. Journal of Attention Disorders. 2018;**22**(10):947-958

[49] Bilginer Ç, Yıldırım S, Törenek R, Özkaya AK. Patients with autism in the emergency department: Cause of admissions and challenges. International Journal of Developmental Disabilities. 2023;**69**(5):710-716

[50] Mulraney M, Schilpzand EJ, Hazell P, Nicholson JM, Anderson V, Efron D, et al. Comorbidity and correlates of disruptive mood dysregulation disorder in 6-8-year-old children with ADHD. European Child & Adolescent Psychiatry. 2016;**25**(3):321-330

[51] Yoshimasu K, Barbaresi WJ, Colligan RC, Voigt RG, Killian JM, Weaver AL, et al. Adults with persistent ADHD: Gender and psychiatric comorbidities—A population-based longitudinal study. Journal of Attention Disorders. 2018;**22**(6):535-546

[52] Klassen LJ, Blackwood CM, Reaume CJ, Schaffer S, Burns JG. A survey of adult referrals to specialist attention-deficit/hyperactivity disorder clinics in Canada. International Journal of General Medicine. 2017;**11**:1-10

[53] Yazıcı M, Puşuroğlu M. Comorbidity of attention deficit hyperactivity disorder in young adults who had major depressive disorder. Annals of Saudi Medicine. 2025;**45**(2):95-103

[54] Kooij JJS, Huss M, Asherson P, Akehurst R, Beusterien K, French A,

et al. Distinguishing comorbidity and successful management of adult ADHD. Journal of Attention Disorders. 2012;**16**(5_suppl):3S-19S

[55] Schein J, Cloutier M, Gauthier-Loiselle M, Bungay R, Arpin E, Guerin A, et al. Risk factors associated with newly diagnosed attention-deficit/hyperactivity disorder in adults: A retrospective case-control study. BMC Psychiatry. 2023;**23**(1):870

[56] Hodgkins P, Setyawan J, Mitra D, Davis K, Quintero J, Fridman M, et al. Management of ADHD in children across Europe: Patient demographics, physician characteristics and treatment patterns. European Journal of Pediatrics. 2013;**172**(7):895-906

[57] Ginsberg Y, Quintero J, Anand E, Casillas M, Upadhyaya HP. Underdiagnosis of attention-deficit/hyperactivity disorder in adult patients. The Primary Care Companion for CNS Disorders. 2014;**16**(3):PCC.13r01600

[58] Siddiqui U, Conover MM, Voss EA, Kern DM, Litvak M, Antunes J. Sex differences in diagnosis and treatment timing of comorbid depression/anxiety and disease subtypes in patients with ADHD: A database study. Journal of Attention Disorders. 2024;**28**(10):1347-1356

[59] Magnante AT, Ord AS, Kuschel S, Shura RD. An evaluation of the relationship between objective and subjective measures of attention. Psychology and Neuroscience. 2024;**17**(2):104-121

[60] Guo N, Fuermaier ABM, Koerts J, Tucha O, Scherbaum N, Müller BW. Networks of neuropsychological functions in the clinical evaluation of adult ADHD. Assessment. 2023;**30**(6):1719-1736

[61] Rommelse N, Altink M, Martin N, Buschgens C, Buitelaar J, Sergeant J, et al. Neuropsychological measures probably facilitate heritability research of ADHD. Archives of Clinical Neuropsychology. 2008;**23**(5):579-591

[62] Fuermaier ABM, Tucha L, Butzbach M, Weisbrod M, Aschenbrenner S, Tucha O. ADHD at the workplace: ADHD symptoms, diagnostic status, and work-related functioning. Journal of Neural Transmission. 2021;**128**(7):1021-1031

[63] Rizzutti S, Schuch V, Augusto BM, Coimbra CC, Pereira JPC, Bueno OFA. Neuropsychological profiles correlated with clinical and behavioral impairments in a sample of Brazilian children with attention-deficit hyperactivity disorder. Frontiers in Psychiatry. 2015;**6**:163

[64] Nguyen T, Xiao E, Clark A, Shamim A, Maheshwari A. Screening for ADHD in adult patients with epilepsy: Prevalence of symptoms and challenges to diagnosis. Journal of Attention Disorders. 2024;**28**(1):51-57

[65] Breaux RP, Griffith SF, Harvey EA. Preschool neuropsychological measures as predictors of later attention deficit hyperactivity disorder. Journal of Abnormal Child Psychology. 2016;**44**(8):1455-1471

[66] Cendes F, McDonald CR. Artificial intelligence applications in the imaging of epilepsy and its comorbidities: Present and future. Epilepsy Currents. 2022;**22**(2):91-96

[67] Wojtara M, Rana E, Rahman T, Khanna P, Singh H. Artificial intelligence in rare disease diagnosis and treatment. Clinical and Translational Science. 2023;**16**(11):2106-2111

[68] Kichloo A, El-amir Z, Shaka H, Wani F, Syed SJ. Predictors of 30-day

readmissions for adrenal insufficiency: A retrospective national database study. Clinical Endocrinology. 2021;**95**(2):269-276

[69] Khanna NN, Maindarkar MA, Viswanathan V, Puvvula A, Paul S, Bhagawati M, et al. Cardiovascular/stroke risk stratification in diabetic foot infection patients using deep learning-based artificial intelligence: An investigative study. Journal of Clinical Medicine. 2022;**11**(22):6844

[70] Frazier TW, Demaree HA, Youngstrom EA. Meta-analysis of intellectual and neuropsychological test performance in attention-deficit/hyperactivity disorder. Neuropsychology. 2004;**18**(3):543-555

[71] Vahid A, Bluschke A, Roessner V, Stober S, Beste C. Deep learning based on event-related EEG differentiates children with ADHD from healthy controls. Journal of Clinical Medicine. 2019;**8**(7):1055

[72] Lin H, Haider SP, Kaltenhauser S, Mozayan A, Malhotra A, Constable RT, et al. Population level multimodal neuroimaging correlates of attention-deficit hyperactivity disorder among children. Frontiers in Neuroscience. 2023;**17**:1138670

[73] Dubreuil-Vall L, Ruffini G, Camprodon JA. Deep learning convolutional neural networks discriminate adult ADHD from healthy individuals on the basis of event-related spectral EEG. Frontiers in Neuroscience. 2020;**14**:251

[74] Crippa A, Salvatore C, Molteni E, Mauri M, Salandi A, Trabattoni S, et al. The utility of a computerized algorithm based on a multi-domain profile of measures for the diagnosis of attention deficit/hyperactivity disorder. Frontiers in Psychiatry. 2017;**8**:189

[75] Chen IC, Chang CL, Chang MH, Ko LW. Developing a Reliable and Practical Multi-Domain Model to Facilitate the Diagnosis of ADHD in Older Preschool Children. 2024

[76] Li Y, Yang Y, Nair R, Naqvi M. Action-based ADHD diagnosis in video. In: ESANN 2023 Proceedings. Louvain-la-Neuve. Belgium: Ciaco - i6doc.com; 2023. pp. 453-458

[77] Lee W, Lee S, Lee D, Jun K, Ahn DH, Kim MS. Deep learning-based ADHD and ADHD-RISK classification technology through the recognition of children's abnormal behaviors during the robot-led ADHD screening game. Sensors. 2022;**23**(1):278

[78] Liu B, Liu X, Wei J, Sun S, Chen W, Deng Y. Global research progress of electroencephalography applications in attention deficit hyperactivity disorder: Bibliometrics and visualized analysis. Medicine. 2024;**103**(38):e39668

[79] Cho Y, Talboys SL. Trends in South Korean medical device development for attention-deficit/hyperactivity disorder and autism spectrum disorder: Narrative review. JMIR Biomedical Engineering. 2024;**9**:e60399

[80] Davis NO, Lerebours R, Aiello RE, Carpenter KLH, Compton S, Franz L, et al. Behavioral characteristics of toddlers later identified with an autism diagnosis, ADHD symptoms, or combined autism and ADHD symptoms. Journal of Child Psychology and Psychiatry. 2025;**66**(2):214-224

[81] Lin IC, Chang SC, Huang YJ, Kuo TBJ, Chiu HW. Distinguishing different types of attention deficit hyperactivity disorder in children using artificial neural network with clinical intelligent test. Frontiers in Psychology. 2023;**13**:1067771

[82] Christiansen H, Chavanon ML, Hirsch O, Schmidt MH, Meyer C, Müller A, et al. Use of machine learning to classify adult ADHD and other conditions based on the Conners' adult ADHD rating scales. Scientific Reports. 2020;**10**(1):18871

[83] Mikolas P, Vahid A, Bernardoni F, Süß M, Martini J, Beste C, et al. Training a machine learning classifier to identify ADHD based on real-world clinical data from medical records. Scientific Reports. 2022;**12**(1):12934

[84] Wang P, Ai X, Zhang X, Ma F, Zhuang Y, Wang S. Evaluating virtual reality technology in psychotherapy: Impacts on anxiety, depression, and ADHD. Frontiers in Psychiatry. 2024;**15**:1480788

[85] Young Z, Moghaddam N, Tickle A. The efficacy of cognitive behavioral therapy for adults with ADHD: A systematic review and meta-analysis of randomized controlled trials. Journal of Attention Disorders. 2020;**24**(6):875-888

[86] Peng X, Lin P, Zhang T, Wang J. Extreme learning machine-based classification of ADHD using brain structural MRI data. PLoS One. 2013;**8**(11):e79476